Sorted

THE ACTIVE WOMAN'S GUIDE TO HEALTH

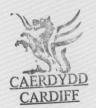

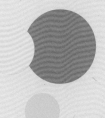

Sorted

THE ACTIVE WOMAN'S GUIDE TO HEALTH

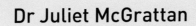

Dr Juliet McGrattan

BLOOMSBURY

LONDON · OXFORD · NEW YORK · NEW DELHI · SYDNEY

BLOOMSBURY SPORT

An imprint of Bloomsbury Publishing Plc

50 Bedford Square	1385 Broadway
London	New York
WC1B 3DP	NY 10018
UK	USA

www.bloomsbury.com

BLOOMSBURY and the Diana logo are trademarks of Bloomsbury Publishing Plc

First published 2017
© Juliet McGrattan, 2017
For photo credits please see page 253

British Library Cataloguing-in-Publication Data
A catalogue record for this book is available from the British Library.

Library of Congress Cataloguing-in-Publication data has been applied for.

ISBN: Print: 978-1-4729-2479-7
            ePDF: 978-1-4729-2481-0
            ePub: 978-1-4729-2480-3

2 4 6 8 10 9 7 5 3 1

Typeset in Glypha and Bliss

Printed and bound in China by C&C Offset Printing Co

Bloomsbury Publishing Plc makes every effort to ensure that the papers used
in the manufacture of our books are natural, recyclable products made from
wood grown in well-managed forests. Our manufacturing processes conform
to the environmental regulations of the country of origin.

To find out more about our authors and books visit www.bloomsbury.com.
Here you will find extracts, author interviews, details of forthcoming events
and the option to sign up for our newsletters.

Contents

Acknowledgements

So many people have played a part in this book, the culmination of my long journey from GP to health writer. Thank you to them all, especially the staff at Dalton Square Practice who have kept me afloat on the stormy seas of General Practice, Christina Macdonald and *Women's Running*, who started my writing career, Shona Thomson, who provided the electricity for my lightbulb moment, Helen Murray for all her enthusiasm, and Lucy Waterlow, who guided me when I didn't know where to start. Along the way I've had enormous support and encouragement from all my friends (I'll repay all those favours I promise). Special thanks to Lisa Jackson, the 261 Fearless team, Kathrine Switzer and Nell McAndrew, all of whom kept telling me I could do it, and most importantly to my family, who believed in me and made sure there was food to eat and not too many late marks on the school register!

A big thank you to all the experts who kindly share their knowledge and expertise throughout the book and to my sister Ellie for her illustrations. I'm so grateful to the wonderful women of Wray Women's Running Club, the UKRunChat community and my followers on Twitter and Facebook for their enthusiasm and overwhelming generosity with their words. Without your stories there wouldn't be a book; you're all an inspiration to me.

Finally, to my little woman-to-be; may you get health and happiness from being active all your life, and by the way ... I love you more.

Endorsements

Physical activity is our greatest defence against ill-health and this is just what we need; a book full of sensible, sound, health advice for women of all ages and abilities. I'll definitely be directing my patients to this essential handbook to help them stay active and keep healthy.
Dr Andrew Murray, Sports and Exercise Medicine consultant and GP, University of Edinburgh, and endurance runner

I've had the pleasure of knowing Juliet for several years. The concept of a book addressing the specific challenges facing women who exercise is just brilliant. There is no doubt that women have far more complexities to deal with over the monthly training cycle. I've had to figure out a lot myself and I'm often asked questions about being a female runner. Having a bible where women can go is long overdue and a valuable tool for any woman. Written with first-hand experience, deep knowledge and sensitivity, this book is a must have resource.
Shona Thomson, adventure marathon runner

Unafraid to tackle even the most blush-inducing topics (yes, we're talking fanny farts in yoga, period pain during marathons and menopausal misery), this book aims to break down the barriers for women who're keen to start exercising but fear there are too many hurdles in their way. Juliet's a GP so you know you're getting really sound, evidence-based advice – but she talks with you, not at you, and in so doing her enthusiasm for the joys of an active lifestyle are bound to inspire millions of women of all ages to lead healthier, fitter and much happier lives. *Lisa Jackson, co-author of the best-selling beginners' running book Running Made Easy and author of Your Pace or Mine? What Running Taught Me About Life, Laughter and Coming Last*

At last, a frank and honest 'one-stop-shop' of everything you needed to know about the physicality of being a woman. Juliet has a brilliantly open approach to all those questions you were too embarrassed to ask. Easy to read, straight to the point and a must on every woman's bookshelf, we owe it to ourselves to be fully informed about every stage in our lives. *Carol Smillie, TV presenter, co-founder DiaryDoll*

Juliet's book not only informs and inspires but it holds your hand through frankly the tougher parts of being a woman like pregnancy and PMS and makes you feel 'normal'. Engaging and supportive, this is a must-read for mamas everywhere.
Vicki Psarias, founder of multi-award winning online lifestyle magazine Honestmum.com

Forewords

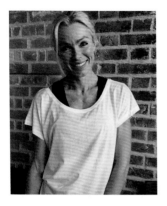

Life throws many things at us and often makes it hard for us to keep active. I've had my fair share of ups and downs with relationship problems, family bereavement and baby blues. It hasn't always been easy to keep motivated and sometimes I haven't known whether I should be exercising at all. It would've been so useful to have a book like this to guide me. Juliet has lived through many of the problems that she covers which means that she can truly understand. If she hasn't experienced it herself, she's seen hundreds of women with it in her many years as a GP. Her friendly, positive, knowledgeable voice will help and encourage you to overcome any worries you have. Juliet reassures us all that many things that we think would prevent us from being active, don't have to. Reading this book is like having a friend to talk to without going anywhere. You can read about all the embarrassing things that you may not even want to discuss with your best friend, in the comfort of your own home.

One of my favourite quotes is, 'Remember, it's always worth making the time to exercise. You shouldn't see it as an indulgence, it's a necessity'. I can honestly say that exercise is my therapy and helps me deal with life. My negative emotions are channelled into positive ones and everything falls into perspective after exercise. I often realise that things aren't really that bad and there are many people having to cope with far worse.

Exercise is part of who I am, it's what I love, it makes me feel good and makes me happier. Women need as much support as they can get and I know this book will help, guide, encourage, and motivate you to be the best that you can be. I honestly wish I'd owned it years ago!

Nell McAndrew, mum, marathon runner (PB 2.54), co-author of Nell McAndrew's Guide to Running

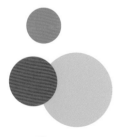

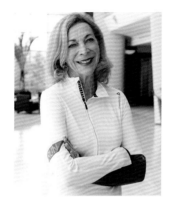

I was waiting at the marathon finish line for Juliet, thinking I'd give her a congratulatory hug as she crossed. Suddenly there she was, eyes dilated, teeth bared, charging the last 100 yards like it was an Olympic final. She flung herself across the line, and lay heaving and gasping at my feet. I screamed, 'Juliet! Juliet! My God, my friend, don't die! Help! Medic! Medic!' Then I realised Juliet was a medic. I knelt beside her asking, 'Juliet! What is it, what happened?' She wiped the spit off her face and grinned up at me.

'I just ran a personal best, that's what happened!' she replied.

Don't kid yourself. In this mild-mannered, calm, frank and attentive physician is the heart of a lion. But it's not a heart that's focused on winning and competition, instead it's a compassionate heart that's heard and experienced so much and wants to share. What Juliet knows to be true she's often experienced herself – or asked of herself to experience – as a medical confidante, mother, and as a runner and coach.

She's been there and knows that the simple act of movement transforms women's lives. All women; all the time. Now in *Sorted: The Active Woman's Guide to Health*, Juliet breaks the health barriers that hold women back. There are no secrets, taboo topics, ridiculous demands or expectations here; instead a friendly guide to help give you joy for the rest of your life.

Juliet's heart is determined to share, and share she does, whether you need an answer to your dark questions or to your lame excuses. She knows more about you than you do, too. She knows you have more spirit and capability than you can imagine. Enjoy the remarkable journey in these pages: find your soul, your strength, your fearlessness. Move.

Kathrine Switzer **Athlete:** *first woman to officially enter and run the Boston Marathon; winner of New York City Marathon.* **Author:** *Marathon Woman and Running and Walking for Women Over 40; co-author: 26.2 Marathon Stories.* **Activist:** *Founder of 261 Fearless, a global movement of women's empowerment through running.*

Preface

It's an honour to finally present my book to you. I've dreamed of writing it for so long. I'm a busy working mum of three children, a GP and a health writer. I've run marathons, climbed mountains, snowboarded and fallen off my bike, but doing exercise wasn't always top of my priority list. I just dabbled in it from time to time. It wasn't until I had my third child that I really decided to get fit. This decision changed my life. It's never been the same since; it's better in so many ways. Feeling fit and healthy is incredibly empowering. It helps us in all that we do, not to mention making us live longer; but more of that later!

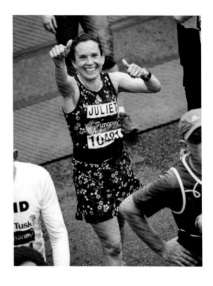

I wish I'd started exercising earlier. Looking back at my life I can see so many reasons why I didn't. I can see why brief attempts at exercise regimes failed, and many of these reasons were because I was a woman. My body was changing, my periods heavy, I was pregnant, breastfeeding, exhausted; the list is endless.

With 15 years' experience as a GP I've met you during all these stages of your life. I can see how you could make it work and how your barriers to exercise could be overcome. Starting to exercise is reasonably easy but keeping it up when problems arise and life gets in the way is so difficult. Once you stop, you lose impetus and getting started again is harder each time; that's why so many of us give up altogether.

So, here's *Sorted: The Active Woman's Guide to Health*. I want to help all of you, whatever your ability or chosen sport. I want to inform, reassure and motivate you. There'll always be problems; hurdles to jump and mud pits to wade through but you can do it. As you go through life I hope you can turn to this book time and time again. With a little guidance, information and advice about common problems, you can get yourself sorted, start exercising and keep exercising. Enjoy the benefits it gives you and your family. It's changed my life; let it change yours.

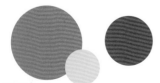

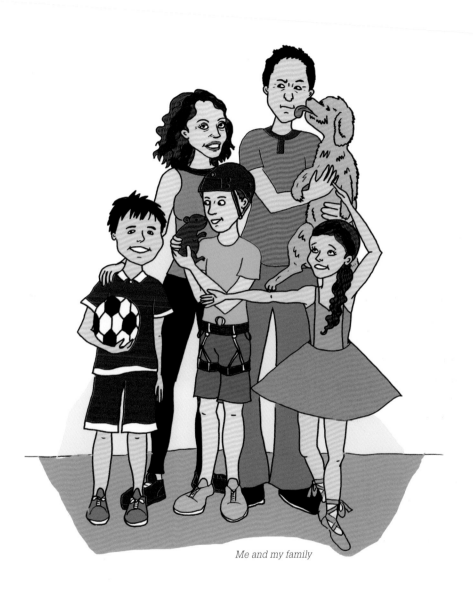

Me and my family

PLEASE REMEMBER THIS BOOK IS A GUIDE AND IF YOU AREN'T SURE ABOUT SOMETHING YOU SHOULD MAKE AN APPOINTMENT WITH YOUR DOCTOR, WHO CAN ASSESS YOUR PERSONAL SITUATION.

Chapter 1

WHY BOTHER?

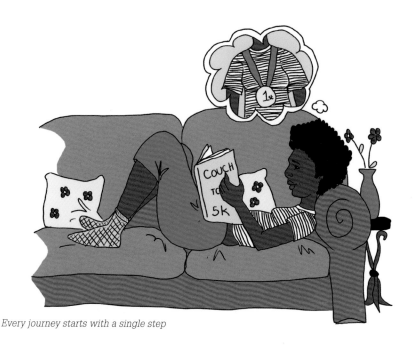

Every journey starts with a single step

Ask people how much exercise they do and the vast majority will look guilty, groan and say, 'Not enough, I should do more'. It can be hard to make time and find the motivation for exercise but it's easier if you really understand the risks of not moving and the positives of being active. There are so many life-changing benefits to exercising; it isn't just about weight control. It doesn't have to involve misery, loads of your hard-earned cash or hours of your time. It's possible to enjoy exercise, for free, and fit it into everyday life. We all deserve to experience the pleasures and vitality it can bring.

We're moving less

We're sitting more and moving less. With lots of us working from home and the ease of on-line shopping, we make significantly fewer journeys than we did ten years ago. The National Travel Survey carried out by the Department for Transport in 2013 showed that each English person makes 128 fewer trips away from home each year than they did in

2002. When we do go out, we're relying on cars for 64 per cent of our journeys, 22 per cent are made on foot and only 2 per cent by bike. Can you believe that 20 per cent of respondents said they walk for 20 minutes or more, less than once a year or never? Four out of five disabled people do little or no exercise and a shocking 45 per cent of women (that's almost half of us) are not active enough for good health.

> JUST KEEP MOVING; SOMETHING IS BETTER THAN NOTHING.

The problem with the sofa

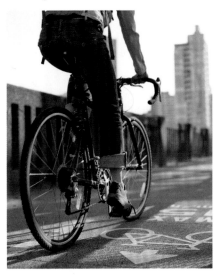

Is not moving so much really that harmful? Well, we were designed to move. We have our own power storage systems called mitochondria. These are the powerhouses of our cells and some cells, such as those in our muscles, are packed with mitochondria. They're continuously working away, turning food into energy ready for us to use. If we don't move and the energy isn't needed, it builds up and is released in the form of free radicals which damage or kill the cell. When we exercise, however, the chemical energy doesn't build up, it's used up, fewer free radicals form and cells aren't damaged. This doesn't have to mean going for a really sweaty workout, it just means doing something that uses our muscles. Taking short regular walk breaks during a long day at the computer is a good example. Keeping healthy isn't just about hard continuous exercise sessions, it's about generally keeping moving on and off throughout the day.

How does exercise make you healthy?

We all know that doing exercise will make us healthier and reduce our risk of lots of different types of diseases. How it does this is a topic of much debate and research, and there are many possible theories. For example, exercise can help us maintain a healthy weight; obesity is linked to an increased risk of many conditions such as heart disease, diabetes and cancer. Some of the benefits of exercise may come from its ability to reduce stress, although this is a difficult theory to prove and measure. Exercise also causes the release of many chemicals and hormones in the body and we're gradually beginning to understand the role that some of these might play.

Exercise as an anti-inflammatory

We now know that inflammation isn't just involved in things like sore throats and twisted ankles. It's a major part of most diseases including heart disease, cancer and dementia. Those excess free radicals in your mitochondria cause inflammation. Grumbling low levels of inflammation will, over time, cause damage, leading to serious conditions. Here's the good news. When you exercise, your muscle fibres produce substances called myokines. These are anti-inflammatories and they whizz around your body in the bloodstream for up to two hours after you've finished your activity. So, a little bout of exercise, a boost of myokines and a couple of hours of anti-inflammatory action reduces your risk of some major health problems. Powerful stuff!

Visceral fat

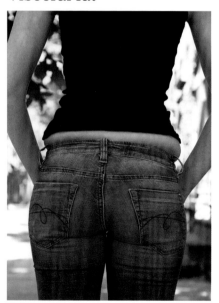

Something else in your body is causing inflammation too. The culprit is visceral fat. This is fat stored around your body's organs such as your liver and intestines. It's much more harmful than the fat stored under your skin which is called sub-cutaneous fat. Visceral fat sends out inflammatory agents which we've discovered play a part in major diseases. Visceral fat also reduces your sensitivity to insulin. Insulin is a hormone produced by an organ called the pancreas. Its job is to regulate your blood sugar levels and decide how much glucose is used and how much is stored. If the body becomes less sensitive to insulin, then blood sugar levels rise and diabetes can develop.

So, visceral fat is not good news. With large amounts there's an increased risk of diabetes and the inflammation it induces adds to your risk of most major diseases.

Exercise is really good at reducing visceral fat. In fact, it acts on this type of fat before it starts working on sub-cutaneous fat. So, if you're exercising to lose weight and getting disheartened because you don't see any weight coming off then relax; your visceral fat will be reducing even though you can't see it. This in turn means less inflammation, less risk of disease and a healthier body.

How much exercise do I need to do?

The current recommendations from the World Health Organisation are that as adults we should be doing at least 150 minutes of moderate intensity activity a week. This means exercise that makes your heart rate increase and makes you a bit out of breath. You should still be able to talk but not able to burst into song. You can break that down into 10-minute chunks if you need to but if you aim for 30 minutes on five days a week you'll hit the target. Vigorous intensity activities when you can only speak a few words at a time are worth twice as much, so 75 minutes is the goal. Of course you can do a mixture of moderate and vigorous if you want. What's important is that you find an activity that you enjoy so it's easy to keep motivated.

Are you an apple or a pear?

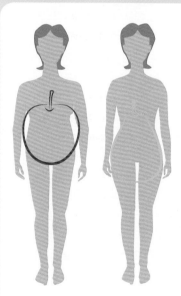

Measure your waist using a tape measure. Just breathe normally, don't try to pull your tummy in. How do you measure up?

◎ Greater than 80cm (31.5 inches) gives you a high risk of health problems.
◎ Greater than 88cm (34.5 inches) indicates an even higher risk.

'Apple shaped' women have a higher risk of health problems than 'pear shaped' women because a bigger waist indicates more visceral fat. Be warned though, this isn't always the full story. We can be 'fat and fit' and 'skinny and unhealthy' and exercise is important for all of us, whatever our waist measurement.

Body Mass Index (BMI)

BMI is a basic calculation of whether your weight is appropriate for your height. It does have its limitations but it's a useful guide. The easiest way to calculate your BMI is to use one of the many online BMI calculators. You'll find one at www.nhs.uk.

BMI results:

Less than 18.5 = underweight

18.5 to 24.9 = healthy weight

25.0 to 29.9 = overweight

More than 30 = obese

It's important to understand that BMI doesn't take into account how much muscle or visceral fat you have. If you're very fit, strong and have well-toned muscles and little body fat you may have a BMI which indicates you're overweight when clearly you're in great shape; you need to be careful how you interpret your result.

The power of exercise

How much will exercise reduce your risk of death and common diseases? Take a look at these figures to find out just how powerful it is:

Death	20 to 30%
Type 2 diabetes	30 to 40%
Coronary heart disease	20 to 35%
Stroke	20 to 35%
Hypertension	33%
Alzheimer's disease	20 to 30%
Depression	20 to 30%
Colon cancer	30 to 50%
Breast cancer	20%

In addition to this moderate intensity exercise, you should do muscle strengthening activities on at least two days a week. This doesn't mean you need to join a gym; carrying heavy bags, digging in the garden or stepping and jumping during dance all count.

If you're over 65, then twice a week you should also do exercises that improve your balance and co-ordination. Examples include Tai Chi and dance.

If you've never exercised before then these are your targets. You might need to start with just a few minutes at a time and build up gradually until you reach these levels. It's definitely better to do something rather than nothing though, so don't be put off by these targets!

Specialist opinion

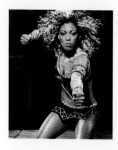

DR ZOE WILLIAMS, GP, GLADIATOR, AFRO-WEARER AND WORLD TRAVELLER. FOUNDER OF FIT4LIFE: EDUCATION PROGRAMMES FOR TEENAGERS TO 'INSPIRE, EDUCATE AND MOTIVATE' THEM TO LEAD HEALTHY LIVES

As a GP I know the theories and evidence behind why exercise is so good for me and for my patients too. I'm extremely lucky that I'm also someone who really enjoys it. I've had so much fun with exercise. I've taken part in everything, from ballet to rugby and even took time out from my medical career to spend a year as Amazon on Sky1's TV show Gladiators. I love that something so fun is good for me and I always try to share the power that exercise has with my patients.

Head to toe benefits

So, now you know how being sedentary causes damage to your body you can start to see the power that exercise has to change your life and improve your health. There isn't a system in the body that doesn't benefit.

It's an impressive picture and this is only the tip of the iceberg. It's no wonder doctors tell us to do some exercise.

We often start with great enthusiasm and good intent but then stumble across a problem and stop. This book will look at the common problems that you might encounter and find ways to overcome them. Exercise really is the best medicine.

Disability and exercise

Women with disabilities often face huge barriers to being active. Sport England report that disabled adults are half as likely to take part in sport as the non-disabled but the English Federation of Disability Sport (EFDS) point out that this isn't because they don't want to. In their research they found that seven in ten disabled people want to be more active. They also discovered that disabled women are less active than disabled men. The benefits of exercise are important for everyone but for those with disabilities they're vital in maintaining physical health, independence and mental wellbeing. The EFDS is a great resource for information, inspiration and support; check the 'Useful Websites' section at the back of the book for their details.

Chapter 2

PERIODS

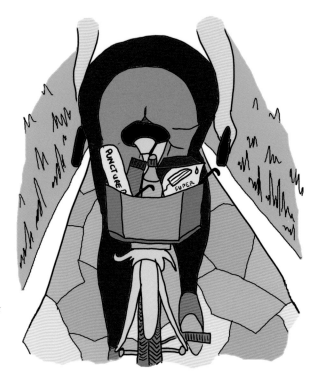

Travelling light

Women have about 400 periods in their lifetime. Our ancestors had far fewer as they spent more time pregnant and breastfeeding than most of us do now. So although you might wonder how they coped without tampons and flushing toilets, menstruation was a much less common event. Discussing periods remains a taboo, embarrassing topic for lots of women. Attitudes to periods vary but there are many of you struggling on, not asking for help.

Periods can affect exercise in a number of ways but generally they're a bit of a pain. They can put a complete stop to it if your bleeding is very heavy or painful. If you're out of action for four days a month that's 48 days a year you won't be benefitting from exercise. That's frankly not fair! Your menstrual cycle can also influence how much you enjoy your activity and how well you perform too.

Let's look at some common period problems and see how their effect on exercise can be minimised and how exercise can actually help some of them too.

Menorrhagia – heavy periods

Some women hardly notice their light bleeding for a few days every month. Others are housebound and end up taking days off work. Between 30 and

40ml of blood loss each period is the average – that's equivalent to a couple of tablespoons. A blood loss of over 80ml is classed as heavy. Realistically, none of you are going to measure this and your period is simply too heavy if you're struggling to manage it, regardless of how much blood you're losing. Attitudes, lifestyle and hobbies all determine what we can each cope with.

Heavy periods can make you feel sluggish and grumpy, but the biggest problem when it comes to exercise is fear of leaking blood. It has a habit of flooding out at the most inconvenient moments. Who wants to go to a gym class with extra-super-night-time-sanitary towels stuffed into their lycra? As for swimming or tennis whites, well they're totally out of the question. Heavy bleeding is particularly difficult for young girls who are just starting their periods. The average age for a girl to get her first period is 13. Periods are often irregular and heavy in the first few months as the cycle sorts itself out, so it's easy to get caught out. It's hard enough dealing with leaking blood when you're a mature woman, let alone a self-conscious teenager facing a mixed-sex PE lesson.

CONTROLLING YOUR BLEEDING

For more than 50 per cent of women there's no cause found for heavy menstrual bleeding and the answer is to find ways to manage it. Even a light bleed can be inconvenient when you're exercising. How you tackle it depends on several factors: whether you're trying to get pregnant, whether you're happy to use hormones and what you feel most comfortable with. The option you choose as a teenager may be entirely different from what'll suit you in your 30s, 40s or even 50s. It's a very personal choice, and you need to find what works for you.

Non-hormonal methods If you don't want to use hormonal treatments (and many of us don't) or if you're trying to get pregnant, you need to look at non-hormonal methods. There are many ways to make exercise and periods more compatible:

◎ **Perfect pants.** Forget those shabby old pants you save for period days as there are now undies designed specifically for the job. Diary Doll are a great brand designed by TV presenter Carol Smillie and tennis star Annabel Croft. They look and feel like normal pants but have a secret waterproof panel to protect your clothes from leaks.

Since having my second child my periods have got heavier. I'm more conscious about what I'm wearing just in case I leak. I sometimes change my exercise plans to suit how I'm feeling but I don't let heavy periods stop me from being active. Even if I don't feel up to doing anything, if I just get out and do it, I always feel so much better. Nell McAndrew, mum of two, marathon runner, loves dark chocolate

◎ **Menstrual cups.** An alternative to tampons, these little silicone, cup-shaped devices, such as Mooncup, fit neatly into the vagina to catch blood. They're ideal if you're away from home as you can empty them, rinse and pop back in. No more carrying endless pads and tampons.

◎ **Sports dresses and skorts.** If you do have to 'pad up' to exercise and are worried about this showing, then don't forget that wearing a skort (sports skirt with built in shorts) or a dress can help hide a bulky pad and make you feel more confident.

◎ **Weight loss.** Overweight women tend to have heavier periods, so keeping active and eating healthily to help lose weight can make a difference to your blood loss.

◎ **Non-steroidal anti-inflammatories.** This group of medications, which includes ibuprofen, can reduce the amount of bleeding during your period by up to a third.

◎ **Tranexamic acid.** This helps blood to clot and can reduce the amount you bleed by up to 50 per cent. It's taken three or four times a day while you actually have your period. It needs to be prescribed by a GP who can discuss the risks and benefits with you.

Hormonal methods Hormones can be used for family planning and contraception but they can also help when it comes to controlling periods. Depending on which method you use and how it affects you, your periods may stop, reduce or regulate. Again, what works for you may change at different stages of your life so it's best to keep an open mind. It can be a case of trial and error, and remember, whichever method you choose, you need to give it between three and six months to see if it suits you. For some women, taking a hormone may be risky so you always need to discuss it with your nurse or GP. Here are the options:

◎ **Intra Uterine System (IUS).** This little device, also known as a 'coil', is inserted into the uterus (womb) via the vagina. It slowly releases the hormone progesterone which thins the lining of the uterus. It lightens bleeding and some women will find their periods stop altogether. It needs to be replaced after five years. It can be fitted and changed in some GP surgeries or family planning clinics.

◎ **Combined hormonal contraceptives (CHCs).** Combining oestrogen and progesterone can be a very effective way to control periods. There are tablets, skin patches and vaginal rings (soft flexible rings impregnated with hormones) which offer this combination of hormones. Used for 21 days each month, followed by a break for seven days, the bleeding during the break is predictable and usually lighter than a normal period. The break can be missed out if a period is really inconvenient. Sometimes the CHCs can be used continuously without breaks on the advice of a GP. You'll need to see a GP or family planning team if you want to try a CHC as there are reasons why they can't be prescribed for some women; these include a history of thrombosis and certain types of migraine. Obesity, smoking, heart disease and a family member with breast cancer can also affect the decision as to whether they're safe for you.

◎ **Progesterone.** Using progesterone on its own is an alternative to CHCs. You can take it as a daily pill, have it injected every 12 weeks or have a progesterone implant which lasts for three years. Many women find these methods stop or lighten their periods but for a few, irregular or prolonged bleeding can be a troublesome side effect.

Causes of heavy periods

◎ Dysfunctional uterine bleeding (no cause found)
◎ Menarche (when periods first start)
◎ Menopause (when periods cease)
◎ Fibroids (benign lumps on or in the uterus, made from muscle and fibrous tissue)
◎ Polyps of the cervix or uterus (non-cancerous growths)
◎ Obesity (BMI over 30)
◎ Endometriosis
◎ Adenomyosis
◎ Polycystic Ovary Syndrome
◎ Contraceptives (particularly the intra-uterine contraceptive device)
◎ Pelvic inflammatory disease (pelvic infection)
◎ Endometrial hyperplasia (thickening of the uterus lining)
◎ Endometrial cancer (rare, and usually affects women after their menopause)
◎ Related to other medical problems like bleeding disorders or hypothyroidism (underactive thyroid).

All hormones can cause side effects. These include spotty skin, mood changes, breast tenderness, irregular bleeding and bloating. Again it's important to understand that we're all different and what doesn't suit your friend may be perfect for you, or vice versa. Lots of these side effects will settle with time and if they're mild, bearing with them may be better than coping with the heavy period.

Other methods Strong hormonal injections and surgical procedures are other ways to deal with really stubborn heavy periods that aren't being helped by the methods mentioned previously. These are carried out by gynaecologists, and your GP can refer you if necessary.

See your GP if: your heavy bleeding is affecting your lifestyle ▪ you've had some bleeding and you are beyond the menopause ▪ you're bleeding in between your periods or after sex.

Exercising during a period

It's absolutely fine to exercise normally while you have your period. Obviously you might have to adapt what you're doing and choose a gentler activity if you're feeling rough. It's worth bearing in mind that a very heavy blood flow can leave you feeling drained and some women become anaemic during their period. This is when your body doesn't have enough red blood cells. Turn to Chapter 11 to read more about this. Being anaemic can make you feel short of breath and dizzy and may increase your heart rate, due to less oxygen being transported in your blood. You should see your GP if your periods are making you anaemic to discuss treatment and ways to control your bleeding to prevent it recurring.

Dysmenorrhoea – painful periods

It's often the pain from periods rather than the blood flow that's incapacitating. Heavy bleeding and pain tend to go hand in hand, but pain can be severe with even the lightest of bleeds. It can start several days before the bleeding begins and can continue

I'm a mad keen runner and periods were just one big inconvenience to me. I'm now on my third IUS and rarely have a period. I can't recommend them enough to women who do lots of sport. I don't even think about bleeding now. Sasha, 39, marketing exec right through until the bleeding stops. It can be twingy, mild and inconvenient. It can be agonising, severe and debilitating.

CAUSES OF PAINFUL PERIODS

The uterus is made of muscle and when you have a period it contracts to make the lining of the womb come away. The small blood vessels within the muscle are compressed, reducing the blood supply. This triggers further contraction and cramping of the muscle. A certain amount of pain is therefore normal and to be expected. It does seem to ease for many women after they've had children.

You can see from the later box that the causes of painful periods overlap with those of heavy ones. Endometriosis and adenomyosis however are more likely to cause pain than heavy bleeding. Endometriosis is when tissue from the lining of the uterus (endometrium) is found in other places in the body such as patches on the fallopian tubes, ovaries and vaginal walls but also on the bowel and rectum. We don't really know why this happens. The problem is that this tissue thickens up each month and bleeds, just like the lining of the uterus, but it has nowhere to drain to and so causes pain. In adenomyosis, endometrial tissue is found deep in the muscular wall of the uterus, instead of just lining its inner surface. The blood shed at period time becomes trapped in the muscle, can't escape and causes muscle cramps and pelvic pain.

THINGS TO TRY FOR PAINFUL PERIODS

If there's no underlying cause, then it's really a case of trying to manage your pain or reduce the number of periods you have, using hormones. There's some cross-over in the treatments for heavy and painful periods so check both lists for all the information.

Period crisis

Norethisterone, a common type of progesterone, can be taken three times a day for a few days to delay a period. This can be ideal if you've trained hard for a sporting event and then discover your period is going to arrive just in time for the big day. However, although it may stop periods, some women can feel bloated and sluggish and may underperform, which is obviously untenable for high-level athletes; they need to look at other ways to control their periods.

I started my period during a half marathon in October. One week early and right in the middle of the run! I still got on with it, rather embarrassed but hopefully empowering any women out there who noticed! Jenna McCallion, 31, insurance advisor

Non-hormonal methods

◎ **Non-steroidal anti-inflammatories (NSAIDs).** This group of painkillers, which includes ibuprofen, is the most effective at reducing period pains. (If you have asthma or problems with indigestion or stomach ulcers, NSAIDS may not be suitable so check with a pharmacist).

◎ **Paracetamol.** Add some paracetamol if NSAIDs aren't helping or you can't use them.

◎ **Other painkillers.** Stronger painkillers such as codeine are available from your GP; you need a careful discussion about the risks and benefits. They haven't actually been proven to be effective for this type of pain.

◎ **Stop smoking.** Studies have shown that period pain is worse if you smoke. Get help from your local 'Stop Smoking' service for your best chance to quit.

◎ **Heat.** Whether it's a hot water bottle or a bath, heat does seem to ease pain and relax muscles.

◎ **Exercise.** Many women find this reduces pain.

Hormonal methods

◎ **Combined hormonal contraceptives (CHCs).** These are widely used to help with painful periods. Bleeding is often less painful than a natural period. Speak to your nurse or GP about using them continuously so you have fewer periods and therefore less pain.

◎ **Progesterone only pill (POP).** POPs can sometimes reduce pain and are certainly worth a try, particularly if you're not able to use CHCs.

◎ **Progesterone injections and implants.** Because these methods often stop periods they can be used quite effectively to reduce pain.

◎ **Intra-uterine system (IUS).** The IUS (a coil impregnated with hormone) is most commonly used for contraception and heavy periods but because many women who use it have few or no periods it can indirectly reduce pain.

Other methods If there's an underlying cause for your pain such as endometriosis or fibroids, there are other more specialized treatments available, including surgery. Which of these is suitable for you largely depends on whether you're planning a pregnancy. Your GP can refer you to a gynaecologist to discuss your options.

See your GP if: you aren't coping with your period pain ▪ your pain is different from normal, becoming progressively more severe or lasting for longer ▪ you have other symptoms with your pain such as a vaginal discharge, pain when you have sex or unexpected bleeding.

Causes of painful periods

◎ No cause
◎ Endometriosis (see previously)
◎ Adenomyosis (see previously)
◎ Fibroids
◎ Pelvic inflammatory disease (pelvic infection)

The ups and downs of the menstrual cycle

Most women feel sluggish and pretty awful for a few days every month. Studies have been done to try to determine what effect the menstrual cycle has on sporting performance and so far most have shown it doesn't make a difference. It's a very individual experience and this makes it hard to measure and study effectively. Most of the testing has involved athletes performing at elite levels only. Anecdotally, many women report low energy levels and feeling below par at certain times of the month, making exercising hard.

The menstrual cycle

Let's go back to biology class to see what actually happens in the menstrual cycle so we can better understand why our bodies feel the way they do.

For most women with regular periods the cycle lasts 28 days. Don't worry if yours is 20 or 40 days, you're still normal. The cycle is split into two halves:

1   The follicular phase. Day 1 is the day your period begins and you start bleeding. Oestrogen levels rise and over the next couple of weeks your body gets ready to release an egg; this is called ovulation and usually happens around day 14.
2   The luteal phase. After ovulation your body prepares for pregnancy. The lining of the womb thickens up ready for a fertilised egg to implant into it. Progesterone levels soar. If no egg is fertilised both oestrogen and progesterone levels plummet, triggering bleeding and returning you to the follicular phase.

Painful periods and exercise

Despite exercise being widely recommended for period pains, there's actually little evidence to prove it works. Many women, however, swear by it, often opting for activities that don't jolt the body like walking, swimming and cycling. Gentle yoga or Pilates sessions can help you relax. Relaxation and distraction plays an important role in how much pain affects you.

Premenstrual Syndrome

You can see from the Menstrual cycle diagram on page 28 that oestrogen is the prominent hormone in the first half of the cycle, and progesterone is prominent in the second. Both of these hormones then fall rapidly at period time. We don't fully understand why some women feel so awful in the days prior to their period. It may be a direct result of falling hormone levels, but it's likely to be more complicated than that. The list of symptoms you can experience in the luteal phase is endless and if they affect your daily activity we call it premenstrual syndrome (PMS), also known as premenstrual tension (PMT). Breast tenderness, bloating and mood changes are common, but sleep disturbance, anxiety and headaches can all be part of PMS too. For many women it's a few days of mild symptoms but for others it's extreme and has a significant effect on life and relationships and shouldn't be underestimated.

THINGS TO TRY FOR PMS

Understanding PMS by reading and talking about it really helps. Knowing what's normal can stop you beating yourself up about your negative feelings. A good tip is to adjust your diary to fit with what you know you can realistically achieve during this time. Plan things that will help you. There's little evidence to prove that dietary changes affect PMS, but many women do report that reducing caffeine, alcohol and sometimes sugar intake can help. Surprisingly, the evidence that exercise improves PMS is weak. More and larger studies need to be done but many women do find it extremely beneficial. Obese women and those doing less exercise tend to suffer more from PMS.

If self-help things aren't working, you should see your GP. Often, combined hormonal contraceptives are used to reduce PMS. Anti-depressants are sometimes useful too and these are either taken continuously or just during the luteal phase. Magnesium, calcium, vitamin D, vitamin B6 and agnus castus berry extract are some of the things you could take to try to ease symptoms but studies proving the effectiveness of complementary therapies in PMS are small and limited. Cognitive Behavioural

Therapy may be helpful if you're struggling with low mood and anxiety as symptoms of PMS.

EXERCISE AND PMS

These six top tips can help to keep you exercising when you're premenstrual:

1 **Plan.** Be aware your motivation may be low so get something booked. Don't think too hard about it, just do it.
2 **Choose your company.** You might be better going with a friend to distract you but equally a session on your own can be therapeutic. Involving children might turn a grumpy morning into a fun family activity.
3 **Pick your activity.** If bloating or breast tenderness stops you wanting to jump around, a swim or yoga session might suit you better. Depending on your mood, a quiet walk or a boisterous game of rugby might be just the thing. The possibilities are endless.
4 **Stop the niggles.** If your breasts are very tender, try an extra-supportive bra or add a supportive crop top while exercising. (See Chapter 3 for more information). Taking paracetamol eases the discomfort of sore breasts and headaches.
5 **Hydrate and fuel.** Drinking plenty of fluids will ensure you're well hydrated, and a healthy snack before and after exercise will maintain your blood sugar levels.
6 **Reward time.** It can be extra hard to get out exercising with PMS so you should feel smug and treat yourself!

See your GP if: Self-help strategies have not eased your PMS and it's having a detrimental effect on your life and relationships ▪ If your low mood and anxiety symptoms don't ease when you have your period and are lasting all month.

Training and the cycle

Despite a lack of clear evidence to prove it, women often find their best training time is in the follicular phase, particularly in the first few days after their period has started. Shorter, high-intensity workouts and races are potentially well-suited to this phase as we tend to feel strong and motivated. When progesterone levels are on the rise after ovulation many of us find this luteal phase a difficult time to train intensively. Endurance events fit well here, as hormonal levels affect metabolism and the body becomes better at burning fat for energy. In the days immediately before a period starts, your heart rate and breathing rate are often slightly higher and feelings of sluggishness

Menstrual cycle diagram

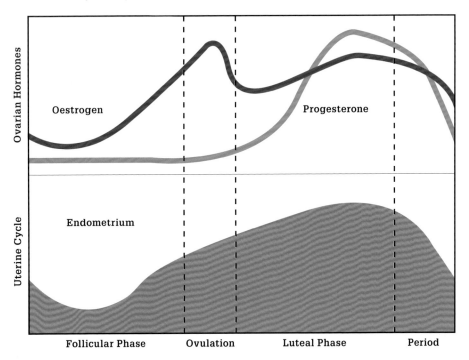

make it hard to perform well and be motivated. Let's be clear about this though, the evidence is scarce and every woman is different; it's definitely a case of finding what's right for each of us.

If you're serious about your sport and want to improve your performance, keep a training diary for a few months. Simply noting down whether you've had a good, bad or average session will flag up any patterns. A more detailed diary could include heart rates both resting and during activity, and comments on breathing, muscle pain and diet. If there are times of the month when you always seem to perform better, then you know to push hard on those days. Similarly, you can adapt your training on your weaker days and choose different activities. But the majority of us probably don't have the time or desire to go to these lengths; we just accept that we aren't always going to feel tip-top, and grin and bear it.

INJURY RISK
Women are more than three times as likely as men to damage their anterior cruciate ligament (ACL) in the knee. A systematic review of medical studies in the American Journal of Sports Medicine in 2007 found that you're more likely to injure your ACL in

the first half of your cycle, prior to ovulation. We don't know if other ligaments are weakened at the same time but if you're repeatedly getting injured, it's worth seeing if there's a link with your cycle. Take extra care around this time, alter your activities and add in lots of strength work during the rest of the month.

Amenorrhoea – missing periods

Amenorrhoea is the medical term for a lack of periods and you should be assessed by a doctor if you've missed six periods in a row and aren't pregnant or breastfeeding. Polycystic ovary syndrome causes amenorrhoea and your periods can also stop if you're underweight, lose a lot of weight quickly (this sometimes happens if you're stressed) or if you have an eating disorder. There's a condition called Relative Energy Deficiency in Sport (RED-S); this is the new name for what has previously been called the 'female athlete triad' where women (often girls) have an eating disorder, amenorrhoea and osteoporosis. RED-S can affect men and women but it's most common in females participating in sports where being thin and light is considered favourable, such as ballet, gymnastics and endurance running. Disordered eating includes conditions like anorexia 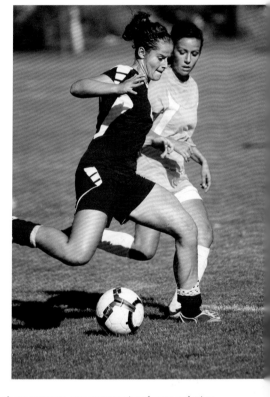 nervosa and bulimia, but also any situation where women are consuming fewer calories than they need to fuel their often excessive sporting activities. Being in this negative energy balance has effects throughout the body such as hormonal changes, including low oestrogen levels which lead to amenorrhoea and osteoporosis. (Turn to Chapter 7 to learn more about osteoporosis.) What's crucial here is that RED-S often affects teenage girls who haven't yet reached their peak bone mass. These years are a vital time for building strong bones. Poor nutrition (particularly inadequate calcium), low oestrogen levels and excessive training weaken bones and increase the risk of bone fracture both at the time and in the future. Anyone with possible RED-S should seek professional help via a GP.

Polycystic Ovary Syndrome (PCOS)

Approximately two in ten women have PCOS and there are some important health consequences. It can be a very confusing topic and lots of us mix it up with simple ovarian cysts, which are entirely different. Exercise can be crucial in managing it.

> EVERY WOMAN IS DIFFERENT AND EVERY MONTH IS NOT THE SAME, SO FIND WHAT WORKS FOR YOU.

WHAT IS IT?

To be diagnosed with PCOS you need to fulfil at least two of the following three criteria:

1 Multiple cysts on the ovaries, usually seen on an ultrasound scan.

2 Signs of high levels of male hormones or blood tests confirming this.

3 Few or absent periods.

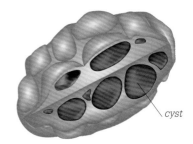

Polycystic ovary — cyst

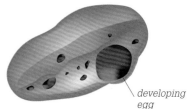

Normal ovary — developing egg

In a normal ovary, one cyst (or follicle) develops enough each month to release an egg; this is called ovulation. In a polycystic ovary, however, there are lots of follicles, usually more than 15 of them, measuring only a few millimetres each. Under-developed follicles don't release eggs, so many women with PCOS don't ovulate and don't have regular periods.

I've found that running has helped my mental health. I was on antidepressants and suffering from terrible PMS. I had very low self-esteem and had become fairly reclusive. Running has brought me out of myself, given me confidence and allowed me to come off medication. The PMS that dogged me for two weeks of the month is now reduced to a day or two. Without meaning to sound cheesy, running has changed my life. Fi Wright, digital marketer, massage therapist, mum of two boys, huge tennis geek

My cycle has always played a big part in my sporting life, right through from competitive swimming as a child to marathon training as an adult. I've had to accept that for three days before my period and two days into it I can only do light training sessions. In the middle of my cycle, halfway between periods, I can fly! I'd love it if races always fell on these days!   Nicola Briffett, mum of two kids and three dogs, heading towards ultra running.

As well as forming eggs, the ovaries produce hormones, including the female hormones oestrogen and progesterone, but also male hormones such as testosterone. In PCOS the balance of these hormones is disrupted. The male hormone levels are high and this explains why many women with PCOS suffer from excess hair growth in some areas, thin hair on the head and acne.

If a scan has shown lots of follicles in your ovaries but you don't have the hormonal changes or any irregularity of your periods, you have polycystic ovaries but not the full syndrome; your health is unlikely to be affected.

We don't really know what causes PCOS; there may be a genetic link. Resistance to insulin is probably part of the cause. Up to 80 per cent of women with PCOS have insulin resistance. Insulin controls blood sugar levels in the body but it also has an effect on the amount of testosterone produced by the ovaries. Higher insulin levels are thought to lead to increased testosterone and subsequent problems with ovulation. The increased insulin levels also make obesity more common in PCOS sufferers. In turn, obesity can make insulin resistance worse. You can see how obesity and PCOS often go hand in hand and it can be a difficult cycle to break.

WHY IS IT IMPORTANT?

◎ Having PCOS puts you at increased risk of developing type 2 diabetes and high cholesterol, and therefore raises your risk of heart disease and stroke.

◎ PCOS can affect fertility, particularly if you have irregular, few or absent periods.

◎ If you have PCOS and get

Beware!

Some medical conditions like asthma, epilepsy and migraines can get worse around the time of your period. You may need to alter your exercise plans to account for this. See your GP if this seems to be a recurrent problem as your treatment may need to be adjusted.

pregnant, the risk of developing diabetes in pregnancy is increased. Other pregnancy problems such as premature births, pre-eclampsia and high blood pressure can be more common too.

◎ PCOS is linked to obesity. Weight seems easier to gain and harder to lose, although there's no evidence to prove that this is the case.

◎ Depression is an important problem for women with PCOS. Understandably, being affected by balding, facial or chest hair and acne can lead to very low self-esteem.

◎ Many years of very few periods may increase your risk of developing endometrial cancer (cancer of the lining of the womb). This risk is still small.

HOW CAN EXERCISE HELP?

The main way exercise can be beneficial is by helping with weight control. Not all women with PCOS are obese but achieving and maintaining a healthy BMI is vital for reducing the effects of the condition. It can often be really hard to lose weight with PCOS. Following a healthy diet helps, but the extra boost of an exercise regime can really make a difference. Reducing weight improves insulin resistance which in turn can have the effect of restoring ovulation; this is crucial if you want to get pregnant. Similarly, reducing the amount of fat present in the body will lower your risk of developing diabetes and keep your cholesterol to a healthy level. Losing as little as 5–10 per cent of your body weight will make a difference, so be patient and keep at it. Exercise can also help with the low self-esteem and depression that can affect you if you're struggling with the consequences of PCOS. Turn to Chapter 8 for more information about depression.

See your GP if: you think you have PCOS ▪ you have PCOS and are struggling to cope with the way it affects you. There are treatments to help with some of the effects of PCOS such as hair growth and acne ▪ you have PCOS and want to get pregnant.

Chapter 3

BREASTS

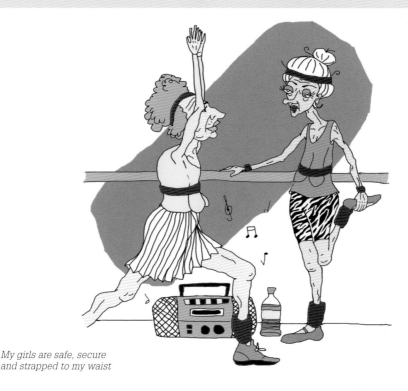

*My girls are safe, secure
and strapped to my waist*

Big or small, love them or hate them, we all have breasts. According to a study
by the Research Group in Breast Health (RGBH) at Portsmouth University, one in
five women say that their breasts stop them from exercising. Breast size, pain
and general self-consciousness can all be barriers to exercise. Whether we
believe they're for sexual attraction, breastfeeding or a mixture of both, we're
stuck with them. Things can go wrong with breasts too, and the startling
statistic that one in eight women will get breast cancer in their lifetime means
you need to get to know yours and do what you can to reduce your risks.

Anatomy of the breast

Looking at the structure of breasts can help us understand how to look after them.

Contrary to popular belief, there's no muscle in breasts. Pectoralis major and minor
are the main chest muscles and they fan out across the chest wall behind the breast
tissue. You might hear people refer to their chest muscles as their 'pecs'. It's the amount

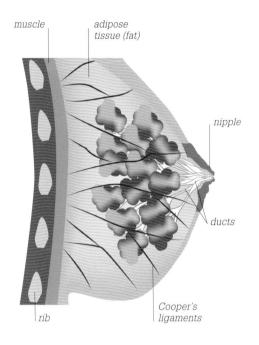

muscle

adipose
tissue (fat)

nipple

ducts

Cooper's
ligaments

rib

Internal structure of the breast

of fatty tissue (adipose tissue) that largely determines the size of breasts. Breast milk production occurs in the breast lobes and there are between 12 and 20 lobes in a breast. Each is made up of smaller milk-producing glands called lobules. The milk travels via a network of milk ducts to the nipple. Within the breast tissue there are also blood vessels (providing oxygen and nutrients), lymph vessels (draining waste away from the breast), nerves and some thicker fibrous tissue. Cooper's ligaments divide the breast up into segments; they branch out through the tissue and, along with the skin overlying the breast, act as a support mechanism.

What makes breasts sag?

The medical word for breast sagging is breast ptosis, derived from the Greek word meaning 'to fall'. Many women worry that exercise will make their breasts sag but it's actually mainly genetics that determine this. The exact make-up of your ligaments and skin, including their elasticity and strength, is coded in your DNA. Breasts definitely sag with age; tissues including the skin become less supple and elastic, allowing gravity to get to work. Smoking has the same effect on skin elasticity. If you're obese or have large breasts, you're more at risk of breast ptosis. Whether breastfeeding causes sagging is debatable. Breasts may look empty or shrunken after breastfeeding, but it appears to be the structural changes that go on during pregnancy itself that are responsible for the sagging, rather than the feeding.

Cooper's ligaments are responsible for supporting breast tissue. They stretch as breasts bounce during exercise. They can get irreversibly damaged by overstretching and stop springing back. That's why sports bras are essential during exercise.

> Two bras is my only option or I'd knock myself out. Anna Cooper, mum of three and landscape gardener

Life before sports bras

Kathrine Switzer is one of history's iconic female runners. In 1967 she became the first woman to officially enter and run the Boston marathon. In those days it was felt women weren't capable of running these distances and when he discovered her gender, the race official tried to manhandle her off the course. She finished triumphant and has devoted her life to empowering women through running. I asked her how she and the other women running warriors of the era coped in the days before sports bras.

'I wore the lightest regular bra I had; no underwire or padding. I just wanted to be modest and not jiggle too much. I only wore a bra in competition and went braless in training when I wore a thick T shirt so you couldn't see my nipples or any bounce. Bras were a torture to us; mine chafed the skin off my breast bone, shoulders and chest. No amount of Vaseline helped. I resorted to heavy athletic tape under my bra but with the sweat, that peeled off eventually. Raw skin and salty sweat are an awful combination! I had scars across my breast bone long after my competitive years. The sports bra has enabled millions of women who couldn't imagine running to go out and run. But a good engineer still has a fortune to be made when they can design a bra that doesn't strangle you, lets you breathe and keeps your girls from that painful bounce.'

Sports bras

The first sports bras appeared in the 1970s. The most famous of these was designed by two ladies, Lisa Lindahl and Polly Smith, who were determined to prevent the chafing and discomfort standard bras caused during exercise. They sewed two male jockstraps together and nicknamed their creation the 'jockbra'. The product was refined, the name changed to Jogbra and, with a colleague named Hinda Miller, a business was created and the sports bra industry was born.

The design and success of these early bras was simply gauged by how women felt and looked when they wore them. We now have the benefit of technology; by sticking motion sensors at certain points on a woman's chest and recording as she runs on a treadmill, scientists can get valuable information about the amount and direction of breast movement with and without a bra.

Professor Joanna Scurr carries out this type of treadmill testing with the RGBH at the University of Portsmouth. They've found that breasts move in a figure of eight direction, not just up and down. During running they move an average of 10cm in three different directions (side to side, up and down and forwards and backwards). Fifty-one per cent of the movement is up and down during running and jumping, but in agility sports there's more side-to-side movement. Breast movement changes as we age too; older women have less vertical bounce, probably because the tissues become less elastic and stretchy. This research information is vital to sports bra designers trying to create the perfect bra. It's becoming clear that one design doesn't suit all and whilst you can currently buy bras for low, medium and high impact sports, there are very few which are sport-specific. Hopefully in time we'll be able to shop for our bras not only by size and impact but by age and chosen sport too.

How to fit a bra

Research by the RGBH has also found that 70 per cent of us are wearing a bra that's the wrong size. Getting the right fit can be difficult and involves trying on lots of bra styles and sizes. I suggest getting a fitting from a trained professional and I've had reports of excellent sports bra fittings at Bravissimo shops and John Lewis.

There are three types of sports bras: compression, encapsulation and a combination of the two. Compression bras flatten the breasts up against the chest wall to reduce movement; they're suitable for small breasts but they don't offer the structure and support needed for big breasts, particularly during high impact activities. They're often pull-on, non-adjustable styles, which makes it hard to find a good fit. Encapsulation bras are moulded and cup each breast individually; they suit large breasts but aren't ideal for small ones. Look for a bra that's a combination of the two, cupping each breast but also keeping it close to the chest wall. Seek out bras with wide, adjustable shoulder straps and an adjustable chest band to get the perfect fit.

Sports bras are often ranked according to activity level; there are bras for low, medium and high impact activity. This is a helpful guide, but if you've got large breasts you may need to step up to a higher activity level than you'll be doing to get enough support.

Underwired bras were previously frowned upon for sport, but now the thinking has changed and wires are used frequently for support and shape; properly fitted, they won't cause damage to the breast.

If you shop online and are fitting a bra yourself it's vital you make sure it's the

I tend to 'double bag' mine. I think they're both compression bras. Anything to strap them down makes me feel happy and secure. Aliya Razzaq, runner, London correct one for your size and shape. There are many excellent sites to guide you through the process, such as Boobydoo and Sweaty Betty. Some have telephone advisors on hand. Choose a site that offers free returns and exchange, as it's hard to pick the right bra first time.

Each time you put your bra on, you should check the fit of the chest band and the straps; both may need adjusting as the bra 'gives a bit' on wearing and washing. Don't forget that bras do wear out and a tired bra stops giving adequate support. Twelve months is the average life for a sports bra and you should replace it at least as often as you replace your trainers. If you can't remember when you bought your bra, then it was probably too long ago and it's time for a new one! Hand washing and avoiding strong detergents will help a bra last longer. A good tip is to rinse it in your post-exercise shower. Leave it to dry naturally, as tumble-drying or a hot radiator can destroy the elastic fibres.

Big breasts and exercise

Breasts are getting bigger generally and at a younger age too. This is partly due to increasing obesity levels, but not all women with big breasts are obese. Big breasts pose a number of problems to us if we want to exercise. If you already lack confidence, worrying about large breasts wobbling around while you move only adds to feelings of self-consciousness.

Large breasts also increase the effort required to exercise; they're heavy! Small breasts might only weigh 225g (8oz) but with the biggest breasts reportedly being up to 6kg (13lb) in weight, the impact can be significant. A heavier load means extra exertion, so if you have big breasts you quite literally have to work harder.

Finding the right sports bra for big breasts can be a real challenge. A study by the RGBH found that fitting a sports bra by measuring with a tape measure wasn't the best method for big breasts. It's much better to use professional bra-fitting criteria. See the section on how to fit a bra for more information about this. Don't forget that some sports tops have built-in breast support panels which can give extra support alongside a sports bra.

Finding the right top for big breasts can be tricky too. More brands are catering for larger women, but there still doesn't seem to be the range that there is for smaller women. If you're slim but have big boobs it can be hard to find tops that fit. What fits on your trunk and hips is far too small for your chest, and sizing up to fit your chest means your top's baggy everywhere else. The only solution is to shop around and try a variety of brands, styles and fabrics.

Skin problems such as chafing and fungal infections are common with big breasts. See Chapter 10 for advice and tips on how to deal with these issues.

Five tips for fitting your own bra

1   Stand in front of a mirror.

2   **The chest band.** This should be snug to the chest and at the same level all the way round the body, not rising up on the back. It should be tight enough not to move when you lift your arms above your head, but it shouldn't affect your breathing. The skin mustn't bulge over, above or below the band. Most of us are wearing a chest band that's too big.

3   **The cups.** These should be big enough to enclose all of your breast with no breast tissues bulging over the top or sides of the cup. There should be a smooth transition from bra edge to breast. If the cup is too big it may gape away from the breast. Most of us are wearing a cup size that's too small.

4   **The straps.** Wide straps distribute weight and give the best support, particularly for large breasts. They need to be firm, but not so tight they dig in and leave a mark on your shoulders.

5   Jump up and down in front of the mirror and compare bras; there should be minimal bounce.

Small breasts and exercise

Let's not ignore small breasts – they can make you feel just as self-conscious as large ones. Clingy sports tops can be very revealing and many women prefer to hide their shape under baggier tops. Finding the right sports bra can still be difficult and issues such as the bra riding up or breathing feeling constricted can be a real problem. Pain affects breasts of all sizes and small breasts don't escape skin conditions such as chafing either.

Breast pain

A review of breast research published in the British Medical Journal (BMJ) in 2011 found that 70 per cent of us will experience breast pain at some point in our lives. It might only be a mild ache or soreness but for some women it's agony. Trying to exercise with sore breasts can be a real challenge.

Breast pain is most common in women between 30 and 50. There are three types: cyclical, non-cyclical and exercise-induced. You might have a combination of these, which can make exercising even more uncomfortable or impossible.

CYCLICAL BREAST PAIN

It's quite normal to have some breast pain for a few days before your period starts. Rising oestrogen and progesterone levels cause milk ducts and lobules to grow and enlarge. Pain usually settles quickly once hormone levels fall and your bleeding begins. For some, however, the

DON'T WEAR AN EVERYDAY BRA FOR SPORT – IT DOESN'T HAVE THE SUPPORT NEEDED TO PROTECT YOUR BREASTS.

pain can be severe and last over a week, interfering with daily life and activities. It's usually in the upper outer part of both breasts extending into the armpits, and sometimes the upper arm itself. Swelling of the milk ducts and lobules make the breasts feel heavy, sore, tender to the touch and often bigger than usual and lumpy. The BMJ review found that cyclical breast pain settles in a third of women within three months but unfortunately within two years 60 per cent have found it's a recurrent problem.

NON-CYCLICAL BREAST PAIN

This is less common but still important. The pain is unrelated to the menstrual cycle so happens at any time of the month. It can be continuous or intermittent, coming and going without any clear pattern. It's more common when you reach your 40s and 50s, and can start after the menopause too. It tends to be in a localised area of one breast rather than all over both breasts. Most of the time the cause is unknown and in 50 per cent of cases it does resolve itself without any treatment, but in a few women it can be

Swimming and breasts

Most of us probably pull out our tired Lycra swimming costume and just hop in the pool without a second thought. Although water itself provides some buoyancy, RGBH research has shown that a swimsuit alone isn't enough to protect large breasts. Some women wear sports bras under their costumes. While this is effective, it's not what the fabric was designed for and swimming costumes with built-in bras are available. Many have 'bra shelves' which are like a crop top inside the costume, but this is inadequate for bigger breasts. Designs with underwires, moulded cups and adjustable straps will give a better fit and more support. Panache and Freya Active are brands which cater for swimmers with big breasts. Don't forget to rinse the costume really well after swimming, to stop the chlorine destroying the elasticity of the fabric.

> I have a healthy BMI of 23 and 32G breasts! Many ladies out there probably laugh at me running past but I simply strap up and get on with it! Jenna, 31, insurance advisor

> I've found getting the right sports bra really hard. I won't wear a fitted top over mine and end up wearing men's sports T shirts that don't cling and hide the bounce. I'm sure I would run a lot faster if I wasn't carrying my breasts around. It hasn't stopped me exercising though, it's just something I have to put up with. Gillian McGowan, 53, finance officer, star of Burnden Road Runners

linked to an underlying problem.

Underlying causes of non-cyclical breast pain include mastitis, where pain is due to infection and inflammation of the breast tissue; you don't have to be breastfeeding to get mastitis. A knock or injury to your breast can cause pain both at the time of the trauma and also for some time afterwards. Sometimes breast pain is a side effect of medications; this includes some antidepressants and also hormonal treatments used for contraception and period control.

Breast cancer is very unlikely to present with pain as the only symptom. Breast cysts, abscesses and benign (non-cancerous) tumours can all cause pain. It's important to be aware how your breasts feel so you can see your GP if you notice any changes.

Sometimes the pain isn't coming from the breasts themselves but from the muscles, cartilage or bones of the chest wall behind the breast. The most common condition is called costochondritis where the cartilage in your chest wall gets inflamed and tender. It usually settles down in two or three weeks, and painkillers like paracetamol or ibuprofen can help.

EXERCISE INDUCED BREAST PAIN

Even if not troubled by breast pain day to day, half of women experience breast pain during exercise. The bigger your breasts, the more likely you are to have pain. The bigger the bounce, the worse the pain, so vigorous activities like horse riding and running are particularly painful.

THINGS TO TRY FOR BREAST PAIN

Once you've been reassured about the cause of your pain, what can you actually do to ease it? Here are a few things to try:

It's absolutely impossible to find workout clothes that don't make me look like I'm trying to be a porn star! It's so hard to find tops that come high enough to cover cleavage when you have a short body and boobage. I feel I have to wear a jacket zipped up, otherwise I'm constantly yanking my top up to stop exposing myself. I have a great sports bra but it shoves everything up even more!   Robyn, horse rider, 5'3", bra size 34F

Those of us who haven't been blessed with boobs also struggle. Whilst exercise doesn't hurt me and my B cups I know it's important to give them support so I wear a good sports bra. My problem admittedly is one of vanity, in that they make me look incredibly flat-chested; I look like a boy in photos! Louise Geoghegan, 47, bank manager, Bolton

◎   Wear a more supportive everyday bra, as well as making sure your sports bra is minimising breast movement as much as possible. You may need to change your bra size during the month if your breasts swell before your period.

◎   Taking painkillers like paracetamol and ibuprofen or rubbing on diclofenac gel can ease pain, making exercise more comfortable.

◎   Changing your hormonal contraceptive (if you're using one) may help.

◎   Evening primrose oil. Medical studies haven't proven this to be effective, but it does help some women; capsules can be bought over the counter.

◎   More radical medication, including hormonal treatments, can be prescribed by specialists. These treatments, some of which are used for breast cancer, can reduce pain, but have significant side effects and using them for breast pain is unlicensed and reserved for the severest of cases.

Breastfeeding and exercise

There's no reason to stop exercising while you're breastfeeding. Turn to Chapter 5 for more information.

See your GP if: your cyclical breast pain is severe, not responding to simple measures and affecting your quality of life • you have non-cyclical breast pain that is recurrent or not settling down after a couple of weeks • you notice a change in your breasts, feel a lump or have concerns about your pain • you notice any changes in your breasts or nipples that are not normal for you.

Breast cancer and exercise

Breast cancer is the most common type of cancer in women in the UK. One in eight of us will be affected during our lives. Seventy-five per cent of breast cancer cases are in women over 50 years of age. Understandably, it's something all of us can feel a bit anxious about, so knowing what we can do to reduce our risks is important.

Exercise can reduce your risk of developing breast cancer; it can also help if you're being treated for it, and may reduce the likelihood of the cancer returning after treatment. It really is a powerful tool and one that we all need to be aware of.

BREAST PAIN IS COMMON AND IS RARELY A SIGN OF BREAST CANCER.

EXERCISE AS RISK REDUCTION

You can't change many of the things that put you at increased risk of breast cancer. For example, you can't stop getting older, change your family history, delay your puberty or bring forward your menopause. You can, however, reduce the amount of alcohol you drink, eat a healthy diet to keep your weight normal and increase the amount of activity you do. You can reduce your risk of breast cancer by at least 20 per cent if you're regularly active. This means at least 30 minutes a day, but it can include general activities like gardening and playing with children as well as more formal exercise.

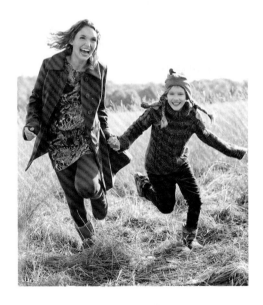

It's far too painful for me not to wear a good sports bra. I'm not vain but I don't want to look stupid, and it's good to look nice if possible. We should be able to love our sportswear as we do our other clothes. Leanne Wheeler, solicitor, mum of two, boot camp queen

Checking your breasts

You need to get to know what your breasts look and feel like. You'll soon notice any changes once you know what's normal for you. Here's how to do it:

1   Stand in front of the mirror without your bra on. Look at your breasts from the front and side and with your arms raised above your head.

    Look out for: skin changes such as puckering or dimpling of the skin, a difference between the two breasts and any nipple rashes, crusting or discharge. If your nipple starts turning inwards or pointing in a different direction this is important.

2   Feel your breasts. Do this however you feel most comfortable; lying, standing or both. During showering is ideal as your hand is wet and soapy and glides over the breast more easily. Put your fingers together and use this flat surface to press against the breast. Imagine your breast is a clock, start at 12 o'clock and gradually work your way around using small circular movements pushing the breast tissue against the rib cage. Cover the whole breast and feel right up into your armpit too.

    Look out for: changes in your breast, such as new lumps or thickened lumpy tissue that's not the same in the other breast.

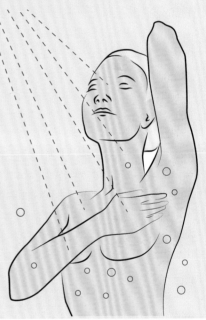

EXERCISE DURING TREATMENT

If you're undergoing breast cancer treatment, it's vital to keep active. Regular activity will help you cope with your treatment by improving your mood, reducing fatigue and speeding up your recovery. How much exercise you should do depends on how much you're used to and how you feel as a result of the treatment. If you've never exercised before you shouldn't suddenly plunge into an intensive programme. It's better to start by just trying to be more active in your general daily life, using stairs instead of lifts, taking short walks and limiting the amount of time you spend sitting. You can gradually increase as your stamina builds.

Chemotherapy causes tiredness and fatigue and you'll most likely have to reduce the amount of exercise you do. That may be the number of times you exercise, the length or the intensity of the sessions. Anaemia is common during chemotherapy and this can make you feel tired, breathless and weak (see Chapter 11 to learn more about anaemia). Similarly, as a result of generally being less active, the amount of muscle you have reduces and this will affect your stamina too. You should just do what feels right for you and know that every little bit helps.

Radiotherapy treatment can make your skin very sensitive and sore. Wearing a bra can be uncomfortable and the skin can sting if sweat touches it. You might need to choose a gentler activity and experiment with different bras.

Surgery obviously puts a stop to exercise for a short time, although it shouldn't stop you generally moving around as soon as possible after your operation. Read the advice in the specialist opinion below about exercise after breast surgery.

EXERCISE AFTER TREATMENT

Exercising regularly can reduce the risk of breast cancer recurring by up to 40 per cent; that's an incredible amount! It's tempting to throw yourself into over-activity but remember that after treatment is complete it might take you six to nine months to feel normal again. Be patient, find something you enjoy and take things at your own pace. Read more about how to stay motivated in Chapter 17.

Lymphoedema

Breast cancer and its treatments can damage the lymph glands and ducts which usually drain fluid away from the arm. A build-up of fluid leads to a swollen and often aching arm. The damage is permanent and the condition is lifelong but exercise can help. Gentle stretching exercises soon after surgery may help to stop lymphoedema developing. Continued exercise helps the flow of lymph, strengthens muscles and helps weight control, all of which minimise swelling. The general advice is to avoid heavy lifting, but some new studies have found lifting very light weights to build muscle doesn't make lymphoedema worse. Whatever exercise you do, build up slowly and stop if the arm feels achey.

Specialist opinion

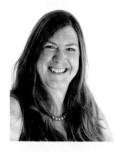

MISS FIONA COURT, CONSULTANT ONCOPLASTIC AND RECONSTRUCTIVE BREAST SURGEON AT CHELTENHAM GENERAL HOSPITAL AND NUFFIELD HEALTH CHELTENHAM HOSPITAL. LOVES WALKING IN THE LAKE DISTRICT AND TAI CHI. WWW.YOURBREAST.CO.UK

Exercise after cosmetic breast surgery

Increasing your heart rate leads to a higher risk of bleeding and swelling, so it's best to stick to very gentle exercise in the first two weeks after surgery to get the quickest recovery. Keeping mobile is important so try gentle walking but avoid anything that causes friction or extra pressure on your scars. Let your body guide you; if it's painful, don't do it!

Swimming is great once your scars have healed completely. After two weeks you can do low impact cycling or spinning; it's good for stamina and requires minimal upper body movement. Running may cause an implant to rotate or move if you start too soon, so avoid this and other vigorous activities for four to six weeks after surgery and make sure you wear a firm supportive bra when you start.

Many core-strengthening exercises involve activation of the upper body and chest wall muscles, so exercises such as planks should be avoided for up to six weeks. If an exercise involves using your arms, the chances are it will contract your chest muscles and should be avoided in this healing phase.

Surgery for breast cancer

Follow the same exercise advice as cosmetic surgery, but it's particularly important to keep your shoulder mobile and your surgeon should give you specific advice on this. If you've undergone breast reconstruction then recovery may take much longer, especially if tissue transfer has been used, as this can leave you with muscle weakness. Again your surgeon should give you specific advice, but don't expect too much of yourself too soon and build up your exercise levels slowly.

Case study

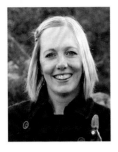

CAROLINE WATTS, 39, MUM OF TWO, UNEXPECTED RUNNER

I noticed a hard lump in my breast one evening as I lay in bed. My blood literally ran cold. I hoped it was just a blocked duct caused by breast feeding my seven-month old daughter. Two weeks later I was diagnosed with early stage breast cancer. My world fell apart. I was surrounded by family and friends but I felt completely alone. It was the darkest time of my life.

Cancer reduces you to zero. It strips everything away. I lost my hair, my eyebrows, my eyelashes and my finger and toenails turned black. Chemotherapy also took my confidence, my pride, my strength and my femininity. Yet despite the awfulness of it I laughed with the other chemotherapy patients, swapping wig stories and championing the NHS for our free Brazilians!

Once the treatment was over, my mind immediately turned to what I could do to prevent the cancer coming back. Starting to exercise was a 'no brainer' and I decided to run. I set off on a quiet trail in the Lake District. As I started to run the mix of emotions I felt at the time of my initial diagnosis returned, especially the anger. Cancer had reduced me to this; a bald, thin, weary old woman. I felt a fury like I'd never felt before. I ran like a woman possessed. For about two minutes. Then I nearly passed out! I needed a different approach, so I signed up to a new women's running club in my village and joined other mums in a Couch to 5k programme. Sixteen weeks later we ran the local Race for Life. I cried most of the way round the course; I was just utterly overwhelmed and thankful to be there.

A love of running was something I never expected in a million years but it's now become part of my life. Like the Tamoxifen I take, running is something I do to keep myself free from cancer. Cancer has taken a part of me away that I doubt will ever return but when I run I remember how far I've come and how strong and resilient I am now. It's made me realise many things, primarily that life is so very fragile. Living through it has given me things I would never have gained otherwise. Never mind this girl can; this girl will.

Chapter 4

PREGNANCY

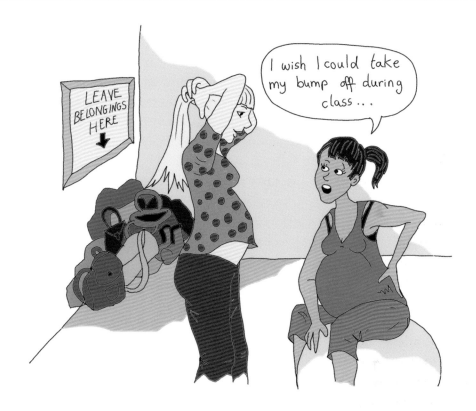

Imagine you've entered into an endurance event like a cross-Channel swim or a marathon, something that will take hours, even days to complete and will push you to your limits. The first thing you'll think about is how to get yourself in shape for the event and you'll start planning your training; correct? Well, carrying and giving birth to a baby is no different, it's a huge undertaking both physically and mentally; getting yourself prepared should start before you even try to get pregnant. Maintaining your fitness during pregnancy will make carrying and delivering a baby easier. It can, however, be a time when being active is the last thing on your mind; pregnancy niggles, fatigue and a fear of harming your unborn child are just some of the obstacles facing you when you're pregnant. In this chapter we'll look at the benefits of exercise and address some of the common barriers to activity during pregnancy.

Before you get pregnant

GETTING FIT AND MAXIMISING YOUR HEALTH BEFORE PREGNANCY IS ESSENTIAL.

Once pregnant you naturally want to do what's best for your baby, so it's easy to motivate yourself to make changes that improve your lifestyle. What isn't widely known is exactly how important it is to take action before you get pregnant.

Many of the risks of pregnancy are related to being overweight or obese, and it's not actually the excess weight you may gain during pregnancy that has the biggest influence on your health and that of your baby: it's the weight you are when you get pregnant. Putting off making changes until you're pregnant means missing a vital opportunity to reduce your risks. In 2010 the Centre for Maternal and Child Enquiries stated that 19 per cent of women attending their first antenatal check were obese. If you're obese it can be harder to get pregnant. It also gives you a higher risk of problems during pregnancy such as diabetes (gestational diabetes), high blood pressure, thromboembolism (potentially fatal clot formation within blood vessels) and maternal death. Problems during and after delivery are more common too and your baby can also be affected with a higher risk of prematurity, neonatal death and stillbirth.

EXERCISE BEFORE PREGNANCY

Losing weight does of course centre on eating a healthy, balanced diet but exercise plays a role and increasing your activity levels helps weight loss. Once you're pregnant the focus switches to maintaining your fitness levels rather than improving them, so anything you can do to increase them before you get pregnant is a big bonus.

Even if you're not overweight, pre-pregnancy is still an important time for maximising your health and wellbeing. Exercise is not just about weight loss; getting into the habit of regular exercise, improving your cardiovascular fitness and strengthening your muscles will stand you in good stead for pregnancy. Exercise can reduce stress levels and increase libido too, which certainly helps with getting pregnant!

Exercise during pregnancy

There's a real risk of becoming unfit as you get bigger in pregnancy and moving around gets harder, but if you're active you'll be rewarded with fewer aches and pains, more energy and a healthier pregnancy. You do, however, need to change your expectations about what you can do, alter your activities and take extra care of yourself.

The same activity guidelines apply to pregnant and non-pregnant women. See

Chapter 1 for a reminder of these. Don't forget, these are the targets you're aiming for and if you're starting from scratch then just 10 minutes walking on three days a week is a good starting point to build up from.

EXERCISES TO AVOID IN PREGNANCY

There are a few activities that you should avoid during pregnancy:

◎ scuba diving

◎ sports with a high risk of being hit, kicked or knocked in the abdomen such as martial arts, kickboxing, ice hockey, football, rugby and squash

◎ exercise at altitudes over 2,500 metres above sea level without several days to acclimatise

◎ exercise that is new to you and requires balance and skill, such as cycling, horse riding and skiing.

If you're used to doing a sport, you can assess for yourself what you feel your risks of injury are, but do consider that some sports are riskier than others.

HOW HARD SHOULD YOU EXERCISE?

Whether or not you've exercised before pregnancy, you need to bear in mind that you shouldn't overexert yourself when you're pregnant. You're aiming for moderate activity so it should make you feel a little out of breath and sweat lightly. For some this will simply be a brisk walk, for others, used to vigorous exercise, this may be a fast cycle or run. There are three ways you can measure your exertion:

When I was pregnant with my first daughter I didn't exercise at all as I was too scared. I ate for two and I put on 20kg. It took me almost two years to lose all that weight but I developed a love for running, spinning and swimming in the process. My fitness routines felt too extreme during my second pregnancy so I stopped spinning and only ran short distances. I carried on swimming and it was great for helping me control my weight but also for my lower back pain. The lifeguards always looked like they were paying special attention to me, especially when I swam 80 lengths at 38 weeks pregnant. I think they were worried about a possible water birth! Mirka Moore, mum of two, blogs at fitness4mamas.com

How to exercise safely in pregnancy

◎ Always warm up properly before you exercise.

◎ Don't stop exercise abruptly; walk around or on the spot to cool down slowly.

◎ Avoid getting overheated (particularly in the first 12 weeks), wear cool comfortable clothes and don't overexert yourself.

◎ Don't exercise for more than 45 minutes at a time.

◎ Stay well hydrated by drinking frequently during exercise.

◎ Don't exercise when you feel hungry; have a snack first.

◎ Avoid exercises where you need to lie flat on your back after the 16th week of pregnancy.

◎ Change your position slowly, particularly when going from lying to standing.

◎ Don't over-stretch and avoid bouncing on a stretch.

◎ Change your activities as you progress through pregnancy according to how you feel.

◎ Always listen to your body and, if in doubt, stop.

1 **The talk test.** You should still be able to talk, so if you're gasping and can't hold a conversation, you're doing too much.

2 **Heart rate measurement.** The harder you work, the harder your heart beats. Taking your pulse and ensuring you don't let it get too fast is one way to stop overexertion. How fast your pulse is depends on your age and fitness. The table below is a guide for the speed your pulse should be when you're exercising.

3 **How you feel.** There's a scale called Borg's Scale of Perceived Exertion (see page 53). The bottom end of the scale is how you'd feel if you were sitting in a chair and the top is how you'd feel if you were doing the hardest work you'd ever done. You should be aiming for about the middle

Heart rate zone table

Age	Heart Rate Range (beats per min.)
Less than 20 years old	140-155
20-29	135-150
30-39	130-145
40 or older	125-140

of the scale when your effort is 'somewhat hard'.

As you progress through pregnancy, the extent and nature of what you can do changes. You need to adjust your activities to make sure you keep within the recommended limits. For example, if you're comfortable running fast in early pregnancy, you may slow to a jog in mid pregnancy and end up walking by the time your baby is due.

WHEN YOU'RE PREGNANT YOUR FOCUS SHOULD BE ON MAINTAINING YOUR FITNESS RATHER THAN INCREASING IT, BUT IF YOU'VE NEVER EXERCISED BEFORE THEN IT'S SAFE TO START GENTLY.

The different stages of pregnancy

The challenges that you face change as you progress through pregnancy. Pregnancy can be split up into three stages called trimesters which last approximately three months each. Let's look at each stage in turn.

EARLY PREGNANCY- THE FIRST TRIMESTER (WEEKS 0 TO 12)

Early pregnancy can be a joy for some women but for others it's a pretty grim, nerve-wracking, exhausting experience when lots of barriers to exercise pop up. It's hard not to constantly worry whether your actions will harm your baby. It's reassuring to know that at this stage your developing baby is well protected from knocks and bumps and if you feel fine, you can exercise as normal.

I'm too tired to exercise In early pregnancy there's often an overwhelming need to sleep and even if you're usually pretty fit you can find you're breathless when doing something simple like climbing stairs. This isn't because you've suddenly become really unfit; it's because your body's working hard making changes to support your pregnancy. Did you know your blood volume increases by 50 per cent in the first trimester? No wonder you feel exhausted. Doing some exercise can be a big effort but it always pays off. You might need to switch to gentler activities but doing something is better than nothing. Exercising early in the day, a healthy snack half an hour before activity and plenty of early nights will help to maximise your energy levels.

I feel too sick to exercise Pregnancy sickness is commonly known as 'morning sickness' but the name is wildly inaccurate; it can last all day and often peaks in the evening. It's mostly due to the changing levels of pregnancy hormones. Nausea is worse when you're tired or hungry, so extra rest and nibbling on plain snacks like crackers can help. There are lots of tips to ease the horrible sick feeling on the NHS website (www.nhs.uk). Exercising can be really hard but a dose of fresh air can make you feel better. Don't forget you'll get health benefits from just 10 minutes of exercise so even if you can only manage a short walk or gentle cycle, it's still worth doing.

It's important to keep well hydrated and if you're feeling queasy then frequent, small sips of fluid are the best plan of attack. If you're repeatedly vomiting, you're at risk of dehydration. Passing very little or no urine is a sign of this. Urine should be a pale yellow and if it's dark orange, then it's an indication you're not drinking enough. If you're sick once or twice a day but managing to eat a bit and drink plenty, your baby won't come to any harm. It's only if you get dehydrated that there's a potential risk. Severe nausea and vomiting in pregnancy is called hyperemesis gravidarum. This condition often requires admission to hospital.

See your GP if: you can't keep fluids down and think you're getting dehydrated ▪ you can't manage your daily life due to nausea and vomiting – there are medications that GPs can prescribe ▪ you have a temperature, abdominal pain or urinary symptoms suggesting another cause for the nausea.

I'm worried I'll get pain or bleeding when I exercise Once you're pregnant it's entirely normal to focus on any twinge you get and fear the worst. A mild period type cramp in the first few weeks of pregnancy is normal, particularly around the time you would've expected your period. It can sometimes be accompanied by a few spots of blood.

If you notice bleeding when you're exercising in early pregnancy, don't panic but do stop what you're doing. If you don't have any pain and it's only some small spotting of blood, then rest for an hour and see if it settles. If it starts again when you begin moving around, or if resting doesn't settle it or it happens the next time you exercise, you should see your midwife or GP. Sometimes the bleeding is coming from the cervix and not the uterus (womb) and won't cause any harm to the developing baby, but you need to be checked out. Similarly, if you experience abdominal pain when you're exercising it's sensible to stop, rest and see if it goes away. If it does it's unlikely to be anything to worry about; try a gentler activity next time. If it doesn't settle after an hour of rest or the pain is severe then you should seek help.

Pain and bleeding can sometimes be a sign of an underlying problem such as a miscarriage or an ectopic pregnancy. An ectopic pregnancy is a life-threatening

Borg RPE scale

Rating of Perceived exertion		
6		How you feel when lying in bed or
7	Very, very light	sitting in a chair relaxed. Little or no effort.
8		
9	Very light	
10		
11	Fairly light	
12		Target range: How you should feel with
13	Somewhat hard	exercise or activity.
14		
15	Hard	
16		
17	Very hard	How you felt with the hardest work you
18		have ever done.
19	Very, very hard	
20	Maximum exertion	Don't work this hard!

condition in one in 100 pregnancies where the foetus is developing outside of the uterus.

See your GP if: you have any pain or bleeding that isn't settling down ▪ you think you're having a miscarriage (because your bleeding is heavy) or might have an ectopic pregnancy (because your pain is severe). Tell the receptionist it's urgent so the GP can speak to you and decide the best course of action.

If you have severe pain, very heavy bleeding or collapse, call an ambulance.

Other early pregnancy niggles It's often the little things that irritate the most. Pregnancy niggles often take you by surprise and make you wonder, 'Is that normal?' Here's a selection, you may have some more to add to the list!

Nipples As your breasts prepare themselves for breastfeeding, your nipples can be a nightmare; tingling, itching and pain are common. The pain can be severe, particularly when nipples are erect, so it might affect you if you're out exercising in cold weather. The friction of a bra or a top on already painfully stinging nipples can make you want to turn around and head for home. It's hard to stop this but wrapping up warm and avoiding windy routes where the icy gusts hit you is probably the best option. Try wearing a softer, padded sports bra and applying some Vaseline to your nipples to prevent chafing. If all else fails, use an elastoplast. Thankfully it's a symptom which usually resolves itself in a few weeks.

Nose bleeds Nose bleeds are common in pregnancy, particularly in the first 12 weeks. 'Nipping your nose' is the first thing to do. This means pinching the soft part of your nose firmly between your thumb and forefinger. Put your head forwards not backwards and don't let go for at least 10 minutes. If it hasn't stopped, then nip it again for another 10 minutes and if that still doesn't do the trick, you'll need to get medical help. After a nose bleed don't do any vigorous exercise for 12 hours; this includes lifting weights and heavy bags, as it might trigger it again. If you're getting a nose bleed every time you exercise, try switching to regular walking for a week to really let things heal up and then have another go.

Vaginal discharge In pregnancy you might find yourself frequently scurrying off to the toilet to check your underwear as you feel a bit damp down below. In early pregnancy this can be driven by a fear that you might've started bleeding.

When to stop

Stop exercising and get advice from your midwife or doctor if you experience any of the following:
- ◎ chest pain
- ◎ palpitations
- ◎ extreme shortness of breath
- ◎ dizziness or faintness
- ◎ abdominal pain
- ◎ vaginal bleeding
- ◎ a gush of water from the vagina
- ◎ calf pain or swelling
- ◎ you can't feel your baby moving as much as normal
- ◎ headache

Specialist opinion

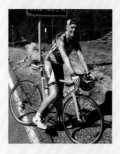

DR RICHARD MURPHY, CONSULTANT OBSTETRICIAN AND GYNAECOLOGIST IN PERTH, WESTERN AUSTRALIA. EX-RUNNER, NOW SUPER-KEEN ROAD CYCLIST AND MOUNTAIN BIKER.

Pregnancy is a great time to reassess your general health and wellbeing. If you're normally fit and active, there are few reasons why this shouldn't continue. If you're not as active as you'd like to be or are carrying extra weight, then it's a great time to alter course and harness the natural changes of pregnancy positively. Some women will have significant medical issues that may be worsened by pregnancy. Individualised care is needed in these rare circumstances, which include cardiac or respiratory diseases, poorly controlled diabetes or thyroid disease. Additionally, if complications develop during your pregnancy such as pre-eclampsia, ruptured membranes or placenta praevia, you should discuss how to modify your activity with your doctor.

You need to use your common sense if you're used to particularly high levels of activity. Over-vigorous exercise such as endurance running can be associated with restricted growth of the foetus and premature labour. I'd recommend tapering to a lower level of activity or possibly transferring to other forms of exercise, such as swimming, in this situation. If you think this may be an issue, discuss it with your doctor or midwife.

By optimising your general fitness you'll improve the chances of achieving the delivery you want. You're also more likely to remain active after the birth, with a greater sense of wellbeing and lower risk of anxiety and depression.

More often than not it's just a normal white discharge that gets heavier in pregnancy. If the discharge is discoloured (green, brown or bloodstained), has a strong smell or is making you itch you should see your GP as infections are common and you may need to have a swab taken and get treatment. The most common vaginal infection in early pregnancy is thrush and there's more information about this in Chapter 10.

Constipation Hormone changes have a lot to answer for! In early pregnancy they can slow down the action of the bowel, making you constipated. If you're taking iron supplements they can cause it too. Try to improve your diet, including lots of fruit, vegetables and other foods high in fibre. Most importantly, drink plenty of fluids; the more fibre you eat the more fluid you need. Exercise can really help as it stimulates the bowel and is a great remedy for constipation. If the bowels still aren't budging, speak to a pharmacist about using laxatives.

MID PREGNANCY – THE SECOND TRIMESTER (WEEKS 13–28)

The second trimester is a great time to be more active as you usually have a bit more energy and fewer niggles. If you've had to cut exercise right back for a couple of months because you've felt so awful, then you need to build up slowly again. It's easy to get carried away and there are a few things you need to bear in mind.

Risk of injury During pregnancy the body produces hormones and chemicals that soften the pelvic ligaments, cartilage and muscles. The most well-known of these is called relaxin. They help your pelvis to open and widen to let your baby out during labour. However, they don't just affect pelvic joints, so you generally become a bit weaker and more injury-prone. Even a simple lunge or squat can overstretch a lax joint, so you need to take extra care, particularly if it's the first time you've tried a move or your activity involves lots of twisting and turning, such as netball or tennis. You don't need to wrap yourself in cotton wool, just become astute at listening to your body and doing a mini risk assessment in your head when faced with a new challenge.

Loss of balance As your bump begins to grow, your centre of gravity changes and you can lose your balance. Activities like cycling or horse riding that require good balance can get tricky towards the end of this trimester, even gym equipment like the treadmill or cross-trainer can prove difficult. In pregnancy your blood pressure often

With my first baby I was really active up until a few weeks before giving birth, but carrying triplets was very different to one baby! At the start I felt really, really tired, all the time. I tried to keep active with basic core exercises, but I just felt too shattered to do any cardiovascular exercise. As my babies grew, my ribs and insides just felt constantly painful. I did, however, manage to keep coaching up until six weeks before my Caesarean section. Jaime Moore, Olympic trampolinist, coach and mum goes down, making you feel lightheaded and dizzy, particularly when you change position from lying or sitting to standing. These feelings can be worse if you're hot or dehydrated. It's wise to just slow down a little and avoid sudden changes of posture. Hormonal changes can make you generally clumsy too. Again, there's no need to panic, just be aware of the issue and adjust what you're doing if you seem to be affected.

> IT'S NORMAL TO BE ANXIOUS ABOUT SOMETHING BEING WRONG WITH YOUR PREGNANCY. TRY TO RELAX AND TAKE EACH DAY AS IT COMES.

Anatomical changes If you lie flat on your back, the whole weight of your pregnant uterus presses towards your back. There's a large vein called the inferior vena cava that runs on the right-hand side of your body behind your uterus. It takes blood which has travelled round your body, back to your heart. If the heavy weight of your baby squashes it, the blood flow in the vein reduces. Imagine stepping on a hosepipe: water builds up behind your foot and the hosepipe swells, allowing a smaller volume and lower pressure of water to reach the flowers you're spraying. For some women a compressed vena cava can cause a drop in blood pressure and make them feel dizzy and sick. You should avoid exercises that involve lying flat on your back after you're 16 weeks pregnant. A good tip is just to raise your right hip slightly off the ground with a pillow or a rolled up towel. This will shift the weight of your bump to the left and off the vena cava, but you should still avoid doing exercises like this for more than a few minutes at a time.

SPD or PPGP SPD stands for symphysis pubis dysfunction. The pubic symphysis is

I'm sad to say that exercise in early pregnancy was impossible for me. I had hyperemesis and I couldn't even roll over in bed without vomiting. Hunger and tiredness made it worse, I think I tried everything! Rachel, doctor, blogger and exercise enthusiast

I was very nauseous but exercise definitely helped. I was told being fit would make labour easier. Running wasn't always possible but swimming helped, and I continued throughout my pregnancy. Charlotte, researcher and marathon runner the joint where the two halves of the pelvis meet. Pregnancy-related pelvic girdle pain (PPGP) is a more accurate name because it isn't just the symphysis pubis joint that's affected. The sacro iliac joints at the back of the pelvis (see below) can cause discomfort too as can all the pelvic muscles supporting these joints.

One in five pregnant women get PPGP. It's more common if you're overweight, have had an injury to your pelvis in the past or have a very heavy physical job. If you've had PPGP in a previous pregnancy unfortunately you're likely to get it again.

Whilst normally firm and tight with little movement, in pregnancy, the fibrous ligaments that bind the pelvic joints together soften and the joints can slip, move and widen, resulting in pain and sometimes a clicking or grinding sensation. While hormones like relaxin are partly to blame, it's not entirely their fault and we're beginning to understand that PPGP is really a mechanical joint problem. It can start at any stage of pregnancy and even continue after your baby is born.

The pain of PPGP can be right over the symphysis pubis, which is the hard bone behind your pubic hair. The pain can radiate into your groins, hips, thighs and lower back. It can hurt to walk, roll over in bed or to do anything that involves standing on one leg or parting your legs, such as climbing into or out of the car or going up and down stairs. Low back pain is prominent if the sacro iliac joints are involved. The pain can be a niggle or it can be excruciating, causing major disability. If your pain isn't easing you should ask your GP or midwife for a referral to a physiotherapist who's experienced in looking after pregnant women.

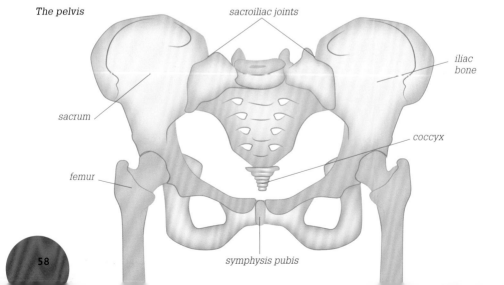

The pelvis

sacroiliac joints

iliac bone

sacrum

coccyx

femur

symphysis pubis

Exercise and SPD/PPGP It's still really important to keep active when you're pregnant if you have PPGP. Some tips to help are:

◎ Avoid any activity that makes the pain worse, including sitting cross-legged or on the floor.

◎ Try splitting activity into shorter bursts and rest frequently.

◎ Avoid high impact activities like running.

◎ Walk as much as feels comfortable and try taking shorter strides. Take stairs one at a time or go upstairs backwards.

◎ Avoid breast stroke and vigorous kicking when swimming. Aqua jogging and walking in the water or using floats are good alternatives.

◎ Keep going with exercises for the pelvic floor and core abdominal muscles (see Chapter 6).

◎ Avoid exercises that involve standing on one leg, twisting, turning or holding heavy weights.

◎ Look for exercise classes specifically for pregnant women and have a chat with the instructor.

See your GP if: your pelvic pain is affecting your daily activities. You can be referred to a physiotherapist. Your midwife may be able to do this for you too.

LATE PREGNANCY – THE THIRD TRIMESTER (WEEKS 29–BIRTH)

Once you head into the final trimester the end is in sight, but somehow time seems to move slowly and so do you! Carrying a sizeable bump can be exhausting and you inevitably have to reduce your pace of life. Keeping active is very important and can really help with some of the problems you'll face. Let's have a look at the common ones.

Back pain Fifty per cent of women will get lower back pain during pregnancy. When you're

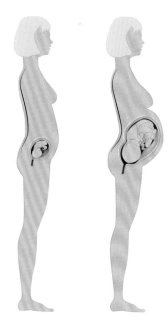

12 weeks   *40 weeks*

I woke up one morning with severe pain in my back which shot into my left leg. I'd never had any problems like this before. I saw a physio and was given a back support and crutches. I tried to keep as mobile as possible and although I really struggled I did manage to keep working. Gentle stretching, warm baths and paracetamol helped. Thankfully it only lasted for four weeks but it was horrible, I've never had pain as bad as that before. Charlotte Peart, GP, mum of two, Scotland

I suffered terribly with lower back pain. The only way I could get comfortable was to kneel on the floor, resting my arms on a chair with my bump hanging down. I wouldn't have minded but I only had a tiny bump and my baby only weighed 4lb 11 oz! Sally Parr, police officer and runner

not pregnant you should have a slight arch in your lower back called a lordosis. The weight of your growing uterus pulls your lower back forwards, making it more arched; this is called hyperlordosis. You can see from the picture on the previous page why you might find yourself standing with your hands in the hollow of your back to take the strain.

Short bursts of gentle exercise with rests in between are the answer if you have back pain. Try to maintain good posture, don't slouch and avoid standing still for long periods of time. Flat shoes are better than heels. Soaking in a warm bath, going for a swim or having a gentle back massage can ease the pain. Maternity support belts which are available from Mothercare can help to take the strain off a heavy bump. Stretches like the cat stretch give great relief. Kneel on all fours, gently arch your back and pull your tummy in and hold for a few seconds, then relax back to a straight spine position and repeat up to 10 times.

Sciatica is common in pregnancy. Pain radiates from the lower back into one of your legs. Turn to Chapter 14 to read more about it out and how to treat it.

Heartburn and indigestion If you experience a burning acid feeling behind your breast bone and in your stomach, it doesn't mean your baby is going to have a head full of hair, like many would have you believe, but it does mean you're normal. Your growing baby is quite literally taking up all the space in your abdomen and squashing your stomach. This, along with the fact that pregnancy hormones relax the valve at the top of the stomach, allows acidic digestive juices to leak back up the oesophagus (tube going from mouth to stomach). Turn to Chapter 9 for more advice and tips.

Breast pain Delicate breast tissue needs extra support during pregnancy; you'll need to get measured and fitted for new bras frequently. Everyone's breasts grow differently at different times so it's hard to be specific but you'll almost certainly need your first fitting at around 10 weeks pregnant. You may not grow

again until late pregnancy but keep an eye on your bra and take action if it's getting too small. A sports bra is vital for exercise and you can add a supportive sports vest on top if you need to. Softer 'sleep bras' are available for breasts that are sore at night. At 36 to 38 weeks it's time to get fitted for a nursing bra if you're planning to breastfeed. Have a look at Chapter 3 for more information on breast care and bras.

Swollen ankles It's normal to retain a bit of fluid when you're pregnant and this often collects in your ankles, making them tight and puffy, especially towards the end of the day. You might find your fingers and hands get puffy too. Use gravity to your advantage and sit with your feet up high (above the level of your hips) to help the fluid to drain out. Doing this for an hour in the middle of the day is ideal but getting your feet up for 10 minutes whenever you can may be more realistic. Rotate your feet to stimulate the circulation. A gentle leg massage can be soothing too. Don't be put off exercise: it will reduce the amount of swelling you get, so keep mobile in between rests.

See your GP if: you get sudden swelling of ankles, hands, feet or face especially if associated with a headache, blurred vision or abdominal pain. This may be pre-eclampsia – a serious condition in pregnancy ▪ your swelling involves only one leg, especially if your calf is red, hot and tender. This may be a sign of a deep vein thrombosis (blood clot in a vein) and needs urgent assessment.

Carpal tunnel syndrome Another consequence of swelling in pregnancy is carpal tunnel syndrome. This is when a nerve in the wrist gets squashed by the swollen tissues. Pain, tingling and numbness in one or both hands is the result. It usually affects the thumb, index and middle fingers, but the aching can extend up into the forearm too. It can be severe and a big contributor to disturbed sleep. It can also affect what exercise you do as gripping handlebars, rackets and exercise machines can be impossible. It will go away on its own but, it can take up to three months. In the meantime, try to avoid the actions that make it worse, use paracetamol for pain and experiment with different sleep positions. If it's severe a physiotherapist can fit you with a wrist support.

Varicose veins   The superficial veins on your legs can become swollen in pregnancy because the pressure of your baby in your pelvis restricts the blood flow, pregnancy hormones relax your blood vessel walls and there's an increased amount of blood circulating in your system. Blood pools in your veins and the result is varicose veins. There's more information about varicose veins in Chapter 15.

Piles   While we're on the subject of distended veins let's talk about piles, also known as haemorrhoids. These are really varicose veins in and around the anus. They might not give you any symptoms and they usually settle after baby is born, but they can cause an awful lot of problems before they decide to shrink down! Veins around the vulva and vagina can also be affected. It can be really uncomfortable to exercise with any of these conditions. Turn to Chapter 9 for advice on how to deal with piles.

Cramp   Cramp is often associated with ankle swelling, varicose veins and low back pain. It can be severe; squealing and jumping out of bed in the night is an entirely reasonable reaction. Cramp is covered in Chapter 12.

Difficulty sleeping   We've all heard the explanation that disturbed sleep in pregnancy is Mother Nature preparing us for the sleepless nights to come with a newborn baby. Quite frankly that's no consolation and I'm sure most of us would rather top up with sleep while we can. A wriggly baby inside you and the gargantuan effort required to turn over in bed and then readjust all the pillows doesn't make for a peaceful night. Add the leg cramps, frequent weeing and heartburn and it's not hard to see why so many night hours are spent gazing at the ceiling. I'm sure everyone has their own tips for maximising sleep but my biggest one is to try not to worry. Relaxing and lying quietly and feeling close to your baby is almost as good as sleeping. Exercising regularly in pregnancy will also help to ward off some of the niggles.

Braxton Hicks contractions   Dr John Braxton Hicks was a specialist caring for pregnant women in the 19th century. He realised that women experienced contractions of their uterus long before labour started. Some women never feel these; others get them frequently throughout the latter stages of pregnancy. The uterus suddenly feels hard and tense for up to 30 seconds. They aren't painful like

I had terrible carpal tunnel syndrome in both my hands when I was pregnant. Most mornings I woke with 'dead' arms and although some feeling would come back, the weakness in my hands made cooking difficult. I never actually dropped a pan of boiling water but I often burnt myself taking things out of the oven. Resting my forearms on an ice-pack before I went to bed was a life saver. Sarah Cunnington, artist and mum to Ellie

the contractions in labour but they can be a bit uncomfortable. Feeling tired or being dehydrated can trigger them, so can needing a wee or having sex. If you get them when you're exercising it might be a sign that you're doing too much so stop and sit down for a few minutes and let them pass. Try a gentler exercise next time, drink plenty of fluid and see if they recur. Braxton Hicks are brief, irregular tightenings whereas labour contractions come regularly and gradually get longer and more intense.

Overactive bladder Needing to wee all the time goes hand in hand with pregnancy. It can start in early pregnancy, often reduces in the second trimester and then returns big time near the end. Hormonal changes and the pressure on your bladder from your growing uterus are to blame for the frequent trips to the toilet. You might get some leaking of urine when coughing, sneezing or moving suddenly. This is called stress incontinence and there's lots of information and advice on this in Chapter 6.

Shortness of breath The extra exertion required to carry your baby and the demands it makes on your body means that you're likely to feel out of puff towards the end of pregnancy. When your bump is large your lung space is restricted and you'll breathe a bit faster and shallower. It's tempting to use this as a reason not to exercise. What you should do, however, is just adapt what you're doing. If you can only manage a short walk, that's fine. Swimming in the late stages of pregnancy is a great option as somehow your bump feels weightless and you'll get a bit of relief, although it's a reality check when you attempt to haul yourself out of the pool at the end!

Shortness of breath can be worse if you're anaemic. There's lots of information on anaemia in Chapter 11. It's common in late pregnancy, usually due to a lack of iron, and you might need to take an iron supplement. Suddenly feeling very out of breath is not normal. If this happens to you and it hurts to breath in, you have chest pain, dizziness or palpitations, you need to get urgent medical help. This might represent a pulmonary embolism (clot on the lung) and is a life-threatening condition.

See your GP if: you think you're more out of breath than you should be. You can talk to your midwife too and he or she can arrange a blood test if necessary ▪ you have any concerns about your breathing, if you're suddenly out of breath as described previously then you should call an ambulance.

Diet in pregnancy

I'm sure you know the saying, 'you're eating for two'. In reality you only need an extra 200 calories a day in the last three months of pregnancy; that's only two slices of buttered toast! You do, however, need to increase the amount of nutrients in your food, so pregnancy is an ideal time for revolutionising your diet. It isn't a time for dieting to lose weight and you shouldn't attempt to do this; we don't yet know if it's safe. Aim for simple, healthy, nutrient-packed food.

There are a few foods to avoid in pregnancy. This is either because they're high-risk for causing food poisoning or because they contain substances that might be harmful to your unborn baby. There's a useful patient information leaflet called 'Diet and lifestyle during pregnancy' on the website patient.info which gives advice about what to eat.

Dietary supplements in pregnancy

When you're pregnant there are two supplements you need.

1 **Folic acid.** You need 400 micrograms every day from when you start trying to conceive until you're 12 weeks pregnant. It helps with the development of the spine and brain of the baby and can help prevent birth defects called neural tube defects, like spina bifida. You'll need a higher dose if you have a family history of neural tube defects, are diabetic, taking certain anti-epileptic medications or are obese with a BMI over 30; speak to your GP if this is the case.

2 **Vitamin D.** You need 10 micrograms every day from when you become pregnant until you stop breastfeeding to help create and maintain healthy bones in you and your baby. It's hard to get enough of it through your diet. It's also made in your body when sunlight hits your skin. If you cover your body for cultural reasons or you're of African, Afro-Caribbean or South Asian origin, you're particularly at risk of deficiency so speak to your GP or midwife.

Case history

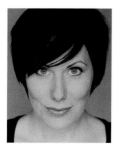

KAREN TAYLOR; WRITER, ACTOR, COMEDIAN AND MUM TO OLIVE AND BUMP

I've been a lot more active in this pregnancy and felt better for it. Despite being an apparently geriatric 39, I've had much more energy, lower blood pressure and gained a lot less weight this time round. Having a four-year-old to take care of has kept me moving and meant no lying in until 10am and no two-hour naps in the afternoon! My biggest challenge was finding a bra that was comfortable and supportive. I'm large of bosom at the best of times and in pregnancy I've gone up to a HH-J cup. Exercising while your giant boobs are bashing about isn't an enjoyable experience but I found Freya sports bras worked for me.

I've always been fairly active, normally favouring strength work at the gym to cardio, but I took up running when I moved out to the countryside from London. I was a little concerned about running while pregnant, as I'd suffered a miscarriage not long before my pregnancy. I spoke to my GP and she assured me that it was fine to continue running as long as I felt well enough to do so. I reduced the distance and time that I went out for but around my 20th week I began to have lower abdominal pain and Braxton Hicks contractions when running. I tried wearing a bump support but it made little difference to me. It was frustrating as I actually felt fit otherwise and really wanted to run. I know it's best to listen to your body and I had a feeling that it was time to stop. I decided to continue with yoga and daily walks.

Exercising helps me switch off and at other times gives me clarity and allows my poor brain space to think. It's helped me during pregnancy and reminded me that pregnancy isn't all about my baby, it's also about me.

Pregnancy and existing medical conditions

Some medical conditions get worse in pregnancy and some get better. Asthma and migraines are two examples. You may find that you have a welcome relief from these conditions while you're pregnant, allowing you to exercise more freely than you're used to. If you experience more asthma or migrainous symptoms than usual, speak to your GP to see if your treatment needs to be altered.

Chapter 5

NEW MUMS

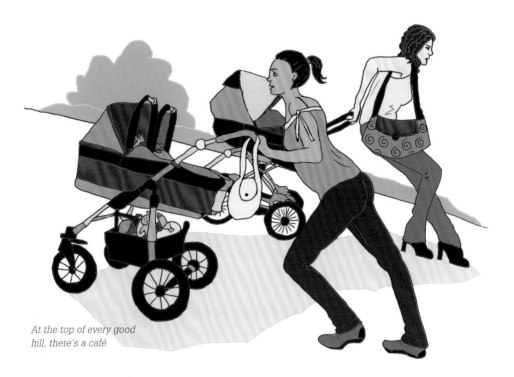

At the top of every good hill, there's a café

Once baby has arrived your days become ruled by nappies, feeding, soothing and trying to find five minutes to get the babygros into the washing machine. Your nights become an endless quest for sleep. It's exhausting and for many women even the concept of doing exercise is laughable. This chapter isn't designed to make you feel guilty, it's to reassure you that the little steps you do take will add up. It's to show that even a few minutes of activity can help you feel better for so many reasons. It's the things I wish I'd known after my children were born. Exercise is actually a secret weapon to help you through a really challenging time in your life. So, feed the baby, grab a quick cuppa and read on (or, more realistically, do all three at once!)

How to return to exercise

The worst thing you can do is suddenly pull on a pair of trainers and head for a run or a Zumba class a couple of weeks after giving birth. It's tempting to seize a random

Specialist opinion

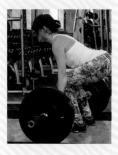

EMMA ARCHER, PRE- & POST-NATAL PERSONAL TRAINER & NUTRITIONAL COACH WWW.EMMAARCHERFITNESS.COM

Don't put extra pressure on yourself by setting unrealistic fitness goals. You need to enjoy being a mum. It's normal to have a 'saggy' looking tummy for weeks and even months after giving birth – don't expect it to suddenly snap back into shape and don't expect to be able to rush straight back into your pre-pregnancy exercise regime.

You should start pelvic floor exercises as soon as you've given birth. They're an important part of post-natal recovery, helping to prevent stress incontinence. Core exercises are vital too. Your core includes the muscles of your abdomen, hips and back; they all help with your stability. Start with simple deep breathing and pelvic tilt exercises and progress to more strenuous core exercises such as 'deadbug regressions' after at least two weeks. You can watch video clips of how to do these on my website.

After eight weeks (or 12 weeks if you've had a Caesarean section) you can increase your strength work. Use your own bodyweight to do squats and lunges initially. You can gradually add weights to your routine as you get stronger. It's safe to start planks at this point if you don't have any abdominal separation (see the section on diastasis recti later in this chapter). Strengthening your abdominal muscles and the muscles around your hips will help to correct the postural changes that happen in pregnancy. Strengthening your glutes (bottom muscles) will also help strengthen your pelvic floor. Have a look at my video clips for lots of routines to work this area, including glute bridges and exercises with resistance bands.

In terms of cardiovascular exercise, you should start gentle walking in the first week after birth. Start slowly and gently, building up to 10–15 minutes every day, although don't do anything too strenuous until your bleeding has stopped. After two weeks your walking can become increasingly brisk. Concentrate on maintaining good posture and using your abdominal muscles while you do it. Beginning vigorous exercise too early may cause your bleeding to start again or become heavier so take it slowly and steadily to start with. If you had a vaginal delivery, avoid more vigorous activities until you've had your six-week post-natal check and wait for 12 weeks after a Caesarean section.

At all stages, don't rush, take your time and stop if you feel any discomfort or pain.

moment of enthusiasm but your body has been through nine months of change and stress; it needs time to recover. Relaxin and the other hormones that were produced to soften your ligaments still circulate for up to five months after childbirth, so your risk of injury is high. Your baby has been bouncing on its pelvic floor trampoline for nine months and the muscles need to heal. If you rush into vigorous exercise you'll probably wee yourself, get injured, have breast pain and understandably never want to do it again! A measured, graded, safe return to activity is far better.

Vaginal wound healing

A smooth delivery without any vaginal tears can make you feel delicate and sore in and around the vagina for a week or two. If you had a tear or a cut (episiotomy), it can take longer to heal. It's normal for the tissues to get swollen and tight when they're healing but it should only last a few days. Keep active around the house and avoid sitting for long periods. In the early days, lots of short walks are better than one long one. Your undercarriage can start to throb after you've been on your feet for a while and when you feel discomfort it's wise to rest until it eases. If it's really uncomfortable then a soak in a warm bath with some tea tree oil can be soothing. If there's any smelly or sticky discharge, it's time to see the midwife or GP, as this might be a sign of wound infection.

Caesarean wound healing

If your baby has been born by Caesarean section (C-section) then you'll need to take things a little more slowly. It's still good to get up and pottering about as soon as possible. Avoid going up and down stairs more than you have to or lifting anything heavier than your baby. Pelvic floor and core exercises are still vital; just because baby didn't exit through the vagina doesn't mean these muscles won't have been weakened. It'll take six weeks for your wound to heal properly so only do very light exercise until after your six-week post-natal check with your GP. Keep the wound clean and dry and watch for signs of infection such as a discharge from the wound or a redness spreading out from it. Infection can slow wound healing. A few small twinges, tightness and itching in your stitches are normal, but throbbing and a tugging feeling is not. Avoid activities that seem to pull on the wound – that includes sit-ups. Focus on gentle breathing core exercises to strengthen the deep muscles and avoid sit-ups and crunches for at least 12 weeks.

It's normal for your scar to feel a bit tender for a few months and it can also feel a bit numb too. Find underwear and trousers that don't rub or irritate the scar when walking. This may mean sticking with maternity clothes for a while. There's no rush to get back into your pre-baby gear, being comfortable and active is more important.

With the triplets, who were born by C-section, I waited until around 15 weeks after birth before I got back on a trampoline. To be honest I wasn't worried about weeing myself; more that my tummy was going to split open! After my first baby I crazily got back on the trampoline eight weeks after having her, as our display team had a television show! I didn't really have a problem with weeing myself whilst jumping, but on a couple of occasions I did poo myself! Oh my word, pregnancy and birth, the gifts that just keep giving!   Jaime Moore, first British female Olympic trampolinist, mum to Flo and triplets

Diastasis recti

I asked Dr Rachel Brown, a mum of two who suffered with diastasis recti, to tell us all about this condition.

Abdominal separation, or *diastasis recti* as it's also known, is common after having a baby. The wall of your tummy is supported by a group of muscles, the outermost layer of which is the rectus abdominis. It's divided into two halves joined in the centre by connective tissue called the linea alba. When the connective tissue is under pressure, for example from a growing pregnancy bump, it thins and stretches, and this can cause the two halves of the muscle to drift apart.

The condition often simply resolves itself over time. However, if the connective tissue has become really stretched and the gap between the two muscles is larger than two fingerwidths, it's worth knowing a little more about.

How soon after giving birth can you go swimming?

If you've had a normal vaginal delivery without any tears or stitches, you can swim as soon as your bleeding and discharge has totally stopped. This can take up to four to six weeks. Don't wear a tampon to soak up blood lost after giving birth because of the risk of infection. If you've had a tear or any stitches, these need to be fully healed before you take to the pool, again to prevent infection. After a C-section, wait until after your six-week check with your GP before swimming. Don't then dive in and zoom off doing front crawl! Take things slowly; try some walking in the water, stretches and gentle swimming first to see how it feels.

Just be warned: if you're a breastfeeding mum, breasts can sometimes leak milk when exposed to water, particularly if it's warm!

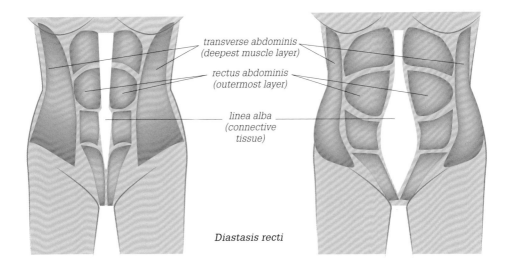

transverse abdominis
(deepest muscle layer)

rectus abdominis
(outermost layer)

linea alba
(connective
tissue)

Diastasis recti

I'm going to tell my personal story about diastasis recti, but do remember my experience falls at one end of a spectrum and many women with this condition will not experience any symptoms.

After the birth of my second baby, born at a hefty 9 pounds 2 ounces, I was aware that something wasn't quite right with my tummy. I was struggling to sit up from a reclined position or to lift the weight of my baby. If I needed to cough or sneeze or do anything else that required raising the pressure in my abdomen (for example have a poo) I had the oddest sensation that my insides were falling out; I felt better if I clamped my hands around my tummy for support.

These are some other symptoms women with diastasis recti may experience:
◎ 66 per cent have some degree of pelvic floor dysfunction
◎ Back pain
◎ 'Pooching' stomach
◎ Decreased 'core' strength

You can check yourself for diastasis recti by using the following method:
1 Lie on your back with your knees bent and feet flat on the floor.
2 Place a couple of fingers under the ribcage in the centre of your tummy.
3 Gently curl your head off the floor and feel if there is a gap beneath your fingers.
4 Measure how many fingers you can fit in the gap.
5 Check again, positioning the fingers over the tummy button and a couple of inches below.

The gap is usually widest around the tummy button, and if you find a gap of more than two fingerwidths you've got diastasis recti. Here are my top tips for dealing with it:

◎   Remember it will get better. Especially if you've had a baby recently, it may well resolve itself in the first few months. If your little one is no longer a baby, it's still possible to improve things by exercising the right muscles.

◎   If you're having symptoms related to your separated muscles, have a chat with your health visitor about referral to a physiotherapist.

◎   You might always have some diastasis recti (mine is still one and a half fingerwidths, 16 months after my second baby) but hopefully by strengthening the underlying muscles it will no longer cause many symptoms.

◎   There's not much formal evidence to prove that certain exercises help diastasis recti but many experts recommend Pilates. This encourages you to engage the deeper muscles, underneath the layer of muscles that are separated.

◎   It's important to remember that other exercises may be unhelpful. Planks, sit-ups and crunches might make diastasis recti worse. If the midline of your tummy is bulging or 'doming' during an exercise it may be not the best exercise to help your separated muscles. If in doubt, get some advice from an exercise group leader before starting any new classes.

Pregnancy-related Pelvic Girdle Pain (PPGP)

This topic is discussed in Chapter 4 on pregnancy, but the problems it causes don't end the moment baby is born. PPGP pain will usually disappear two weeks after delivery. It's safe to do gentle exercise when this is the case but avoid any activities that seem to trigger it again. Concentrate on pelvic and core muscle strengthening exercises and gentle walking. Try to keep your weight central over your pelvis, so avoid carrying your baby on your hip or slinging the hefty car seat over one arm. Avoid uneven stresses on the pelvic joints by lifting any weights, including baby, with two hands in front of you. If you've had lots of problems with PPGP during pregnancy, you should avoid vigorous exercise for about three months. PPGP is a mechanical problem not purely due to hormonal changes, so for some women the pain can go on for many months after giving birth. This is thankfully unusual, but if your pain is persisting for longer than three weeks then see your GP or physiotherapist.

Exercising as a new mum

When most of your choices are determined by the needs of your baby, carving out a short time for yourself to have fun and get moving is vital. Regular exercise will make you feel good about yourself, calmer, more in control and therefore better equipped to

IF YOU'VE HAD PPGP IN PREGNANCY THEN YOU'RE LIKELY TO GET IT AGAIN IN ANY SUBSEQUENT PREGNANCIES. GETTING YOURSELF AS FIT AND HEALTHY AS POSSIBLE BETWEEN PREGNANCIES WILL MINIMISE THE RISK OF IT RETURNING, OR REDUCE ITS SEVERITY.

cope with the demands of being a mum. Using exercise to spend time with friends and meet other mums is a great way of gaining support and having a laugh while you do it. There's the added side effect that you'll find it easier to get back to your pre-baby shape if that's a priority for you. This is particularly important if you're thinking of having another baby as the risks of pregnancy increase if you're overweight.

It's natural once you have dependents to start worrying about what would happen to them if you weren't around. There's no doubt that women who exercise regularly have a longer lifespan and a lower incidence of disease than those who are inactive. Thinking about your long-term health can be a great motivator. It's also really brilliant to be a role model, set an example to your children and let them grow up with exercise as a normal part of their daily lives. They're never too young and you're never too old to start!

EXERCISING WITH BABY

Finding the time to exercise can be your biggest challenge but there are always solutions. Exercising with your baby is one of them. Striding out with the pram or baby sling is great. When babies are young they'll most likely sleep while in motion but soon enough they'll want to sit up and gaze at the world around them. This can become an activity that you can enjoy together for many years; there are ducks to be fed and play areas to explore. Brisk walking is excellent exercise but why not think about running with the buggy too? Once your baby is six months old and has good head control then 30 seconds of running at a time is a great place to start and it's surprisingly easy to build up from there.

Babies that can sit up by themselves (around six months old) can be carried in specially designed baby backpacks. Some babies love these as they're high up and can see all around them. Baby's weight is well distributed and the straps well padded, so they're comfortable to use. It leaves you with two hands free for opening gates, skimming stones and holding the hands of any siblings. Try different models and look for one that can be adjusted as baby grows. If you're using the carrier

Specialist opinion

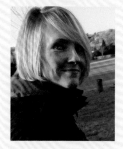

EMMA BROCKWELL (PHYSIOMUM), WOMEN'S HEALTH
PHYSIOTHERAPIST, LONDON BRIDGE HOSPITAL. ALSO FOUND AT WWW.
PHYSIOMUM.CO.UK, RUNNING OR HOME WITH TWO CHILDREN

Running with a buggy

Information on running with a buggy is hard to find but there
are important considerations to minimise the risk of injury to
baby and yourself.

What to look for in a running buggy   Many buggies have sport or jogging in their titles but it
doesn't necessarily mean they're designed for that purpose. The more a buggy has been
adapted for running, the less versatile it will be for day-to-day use; worth considering if you're
just doing the odd run.

◎ Most running buggies have three wheels. The wheels should be large (ideally 40cm/16
   inches or more), have pneumatic tyres and a fixed front wheel for uneven ground.

◎ Make sure the buggy has rear-wheel suspension and a padded seat to help protect your
   baby's spine.

◎ Look for a light buggy. Does the design allow you to run unhindered with a full stride?
   It should be easy to push and steer with one or both hands.

◎ The buggy should have a handlebar brake and wrist strap, crucial for those fast and
   downhill parts of your run. A five-point harness that's fully adjustable and secure is
   also essential.

Posture and form   Keep good form behind the wheel to avoid injury. Don't stand upright, lean
forwards, bending from the hips. Keep your head up, your shoulders back and down; lead with
your chest. Maintain a slight bend in your elbows, keep your wrists straight and stay as close to
the buggy as you can. Running with a buggy will prevent your natural arm swing. If you use one
hand be sure to swap hands regularly to work both sides.

The earliest you should consider running with a buggy is six months after giving birth
because it's demanding and places great stress on areas of your body that are weakened by
pregnancy. It takes six months for your baby to develop adequate spine strength to be safe
in a buggy anyway. If you've had a C-section or a vaginal tear it may take longer for you or your
pelvic floor to be ready. If you've had issues with PPGP, lower back pain, pelvic organ prolapse or
diastasis recti then it's a good idea to check with a woman's health physio that you're fit to run.

> IT'S ALWAYS WORTH MAKING THE TIME TO EXERCISE. YOU SHOULDN'T SEE IT AS AN INDULGENCE. IT'S A NECESSITY.

regularly the extra load will increase gradually but be careful if you're suddenly using a backpack for a heavy baby for the first time. If you've suffered with pelvic or back pain in pregnancy, then backpacks may put too much strain on your muscles and joints.

What about bikes? There are loads of ways to transport babies by bicycle. Front seats that go between the handlebars, rear seats and bike trailers. None of them are sold as suitable for newborns but the months fly by and before you know it your baby will be able to sit up unaided, wear a bike helmet and use one of these methods. The age this happens at varies with the development of each child and the specifications of the seat but 9–12 months old is a guide. Bike trailers and 'box bikes' can hold all your baby-changing kit as well as your shopping and more than one child. You might feel happier on cycle paths and quiet roads than busy commuter routes but there are many adventures to be had by bike.

Look out for postnatal exercise classes, mum and baby swimming and yoga classes. There's more on offer than you may realise! Don't forget that you don't have to leave the house to exercise. There are exercise DVDs, online classes and YouTube clips. From gentle Pilates to sweat-inducing high-intensity workouts, there's a great range of resources out there to help you. A quick 15 minutes while baby is sleeping or playing next to you is all you need. Why not borrow an exercise bike for a while? Seizing short opportunities throughout the day may be all you can manage but it's enough. Great progress comes from small steps.

Exercising without baby

You might prefer to exercise without your baby. There's lots of ways this can be achieved from leaving baby with partners, family members or baby sitters to doing 'baby relays' with friends. Many gyms and sports centres offer crèches and supervised play so you can exercise while your baby is being looked after. An hour's exercise class can leave you feeling energised and in a great mood even if you went in as an exhausted wreck. You shouldn't feel guilty about using these services, you should embrace them. Why not use the time to try something new?

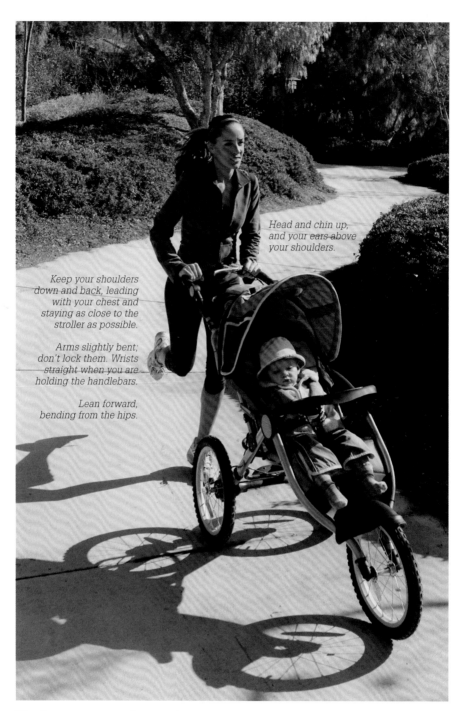

Head and chin up, and your ears above your shoulders.

Keep your shoulders down and back, leading with your chest and staying as close to the stroller as possible.

Arms slightly bent; don't lock them. Wrists straight when you are holding the handlebars.

Lean forward, bending from the hips.

Tips for your posture when running with your buggy

Breastfeeding and exercise

Breastfeeding is entirely compatible with exercise. Here are some tips to help you combine the two:

◎ **Feed baby before exercise.** This will reduce the size and weight of your breasts as much as possible and stop you worrying that baby will be screaming for food while you're out.

◎ **Consider expressing before exercise if baby is asleep or not hungry.** This means there's milk there for your baby-minder to give. Admittedly not every baby will take milk from a bottle, and some people prefer that they don't.

◎ **Wear the most supportive sports bra you can get.** Getting re-measured once breastfeeding is established is a good idea. Breasts do fill up and grow between feeds so you might need a couple of bras in different sizes to accommodate this. Don't forget to leave space for breast pads.

◎ **Protecting your nipples is important;** they can get sore and cracked, and can bleed when you're breastfeeding. Salty sweat running over these and the added friction from exercise isn't a good combination. The Breastfeeding Network advise that Vaseline is safe to use while feeding but a shower after exercise will wash off any petroleum products. If you're concerned about this then lanolin creams are a good, although more expensive, alternative.

When you have a child people tell you that you'll be tired, but I had no idea how tired. In those first few months, I could barely summon up the energy to run myself a bath let alone run around the park. So, at first, it seemed easier to just do nothing. Of course, it's a catch 22 because the less exercise you do, the more tired you feel. Then I realised walking and hills were the answer. Every day, I tried to walk for at least two hours while my daughter slept in her buggy, up the steepest routes I could find. It made a huge difference to my fitness and energy levels. Now she's older, I shoehorn as much activity into my everyday living as I can. I power walk while she whizzes alongside on her scooter, I climb trees with her – heck, I've even been known to crawl through tunnels at soft-play centres. OK, so it's not a 60-minute run or a hard-core spinning class, but small amounts of activity throughout the day all add up, especially when you do them with gusto. Nicola Down, leading health and wellbeing journalist and mum to Daisy

Top tips for starting to exercise after childbirth

◎ Plan your exercise, write it in the diary and make it a priority.
◎ Make sure you've done the core and pelvic floor strengthening before you progress to more vigorous exercise.
◎ Don't exercise on an empty stomach: eat something an hour or two beforehand.
◎ Drink plenty before, during and after exercise.
◎ Take things slowly. Warm up well, don't get carried away. It's easy to get injured.
◎ Stop if you feel lightheaded, dizzy or have any pain in your pelvis or stitches.
◎ Try to make time to do some stretches after exercise or later in the day after a warm bath.
◎ Set yourself little targets to keep you motivated and plan a treat for yourself when you reach them.

◎ **Experiment with different breast pads.** You might not be a 'leaker' but being away from your baby, especially when a feed is due, can result in unmistakable wet patches on your T-shirt. Some breast pads have adhesive strips to help keep them in place. Try washable pads too: they can be softer, cost effective and you can throw them in the washing machine with your kit.

◎ **Squeeze it in.** In reality many women can't disappear off for an hour or two if they have a baby who likes to feed frequently and unpredictably. Remember you can have a great workout in only 20 minutes. Why not take your baby with you? A power walk with the pram and a feed stop on a park bench might suit you both.

◎ **Drink up.** Producing breast milk is a thirsty business and your fluid requirements shoot up if you've been sweating and exerting yourself.

NUTRITION DURING BREASTFEEDING

All the good eating habits you adopted during pregnancy need to continue. Eat a sensible, healthy diet focusing on quality not quantity. Take care not to gorge on junk when your appetite is raging. Eating healthy snacks in between three main meals should be your goal.

Mother Nature will ensure your breast milk is of good quality, but you need to take responsibility for your diet and make sure there are enough nutrients left over to keep you healthy too. It's easy to become iron-deficient when you're breastfeeding because pregnancy depletes your stores. Turn to Chapter 11 to read the 'Eating for Iron' tips.

Case history

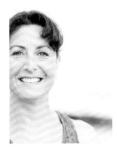

JENNIE EDMONDSON, PERSONAL TRAINER AND FOUNDER
OF PRAMPOWER AND GO HEALTH AND FITNESS
WWW.GOHEALTHANDFITNESS.CO.UK

I learnt the hard way! I trained through both of my pregnancies
and I was super keen to get going again as soon as my baby was
born; not for weight loss but for sanity! I returned to high-impact
exercise after only four weeks, which in hindsight was really too soon. I'd spent barely any
time working on core strength and stability; I kind of figured it would sort itself out. I fell
pregnant again five months later, thought I was fully recovered and had no issues. It wasn't
until I studied as a personal trainer five years later that I realised I still had nearly a three-
finger width abdominal separation which was a major cause of the lower back pain I was
experiencing. I realised how important it was to return to exercise in the correct way. I set up
a group called PramPower to help women do this. I wanted to give new mums a chance to
train without the need for childcare and realise that any walk can be turned into a workout.

Exercising in a group is so beneficial. It gets us out of the house: if we've said to the gang
we're coming, then we're more likely to get there. We get to socialise and share all our woes
and joys (no subject is taboo!). We learn that all the other mums are going through the same
issues as us. We help each other out. If a baby is crying, needs a nappy change or needs
feeding, we take turns in helping and exercising! Toddlers are welcome and they join in too
showing them that exercise is normal, just part of life, like cleaning your teeth!

Carry on taking the vitamin D supplement that you took in pregnancy; you'll continue to
need 10 micrograms a day until you stop breastfeeding.

Post-natal depression (PND)

Most women will experience some feelings of low mood and tearfulness for a couple of
weeks after their baby is born. Aptly named the 'baby blues', this is normal and nothing
to worry about. It's due to altering hormone levels in your body in addition to a life-
changing event and extreme fatigue. For some women, however, the blues don't seem to
lift. You can feel like a black cloud is hanging over you. You've just had a beautiful baby,
so why don't you feel happy?

PND affects one in 10 women, so it's really common. It's more likely to happen if you've had any depression before or during pregnancy. It's also more common in teenagers or in women with other stresses in life such as housing or financial problems. It can start suddenly or gradually, usually within six weeks of having a baby, but it can be as much as six months later.

You can experience a whole range of symptoms such as crying at the drop of a hat or doubting your ability to look after your baby. From feelings of anxiety and panic to guilt and despair, it can be a confusing and lonely time. Some feelings are frightening and very hard to discuss. You might have thoughts about harming yourself or your baby; it doesn't mean that you're going to do it, but it's vital that you speak to your health visitor or GP. Admitting there's a problem is the first step. With help and support you will get better and enjoy life again.

TREATMENTS FOR POSTNATAL DEPRESSION

There are lots of treatments for PND. Talking and behavioural therapies are an effective way to lift the heavy burden. Discovering why you feel like you do and looking at ways to change this is a lifelong skill that you can turn to repeatedly in years to come. You should talk to your GP about whether anti-depressants might help too.

A crucial part of getting better involves what you do to help yourself. There are lots of self-care tips in Chapter 8. Self-care is really hard at a time like this because depression can make you feel tired, lacking in confidence and unmotivated. Just getting up and tending to the needs of your baby can feel like an overwhelming task. The charity Mind has a section on PND on their website (www.mind.org.uk). It gives lots of advice about self-care. Don't be afraid to ask for help.

Breastfeeding and sports supplements

Most sports drinks and gels for endurance sports can be used safely in breastfeeding. It's sensible to avoid those containing caffeine as the dose can be quite large; there's often caffeine in cola-flavoured products. If you're in doubt as to whether a product is suitable for use while breastfeeding, contact the company and ask them.

Case history

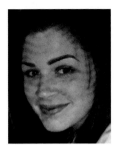

BECKI GERRARD; BECKI AND HER SISTER LOUISE SET UP MUMBALL TO ENCOURAGE MORE WOMEN TO PLAY FOOTBALL, HELP THEM EXERCISE AND PROVIDE A FRIENDLY, FUN WAY TO MEET OTHER WOMEN. WWW.MUMBALL.COM

When I had my first child Joseph he was whisked away to the neo-natal unit within hours of birth due to an infection. I feel I missed out on crucial bonding and I struggled with this for the next two years. I felt he hated me; that everybody hated me. I was paranoid and anxious; walking round a supermarket would have me on the verge of a panic attack. I also got very angry; arguing with my partner over very small things. I found it hard to admit I needed help but when I started to have suicidal thoughts I went to the GP. I was offered anti-depressants but I was worried about addiction and I really believed I could get better myself, without medication.

I've played football for years, playing for various local teams. I stopped when I left school and I only started up again at the age of 23 because my sister begged me to join a team with her. It's been one of the best things that's happened to me. Before joining I was just 'Mummy' who was sad and angry most of the time, then all of a sudden I was back to being Becki who could talk about things other than kids. I had a whole new group of friends and I'd look forward to the training sessions and matches. Without even realising it, my depression lifted. On a bad day I'd go to football, get my frustration out on the pitch and come home smiling.

I'd recommend any type of exercise (especially a team sport) if you're suffering with depression. I started just for fun, I really didn't expect it to change my life!

EXERCISE AND PND

Exercise releases endorphins, your body's own 'happy hormones', which help to treat and prevent post-natal depression and ease stress and anxiety. Just a few minutes walking in the fresh air can help to clear your head. You might prefer to exercise on your own, but joining a group activity will not only give you the benefits of exercise but powerful emotional support and motivation from other women too. Turn to Chapter 17 for lots of advice and tips.

See your GP if: you think you might have post-natal depression or your health visitor has suggested that you make an appointment.

Chapter 6

THE PELVIC FLOOR

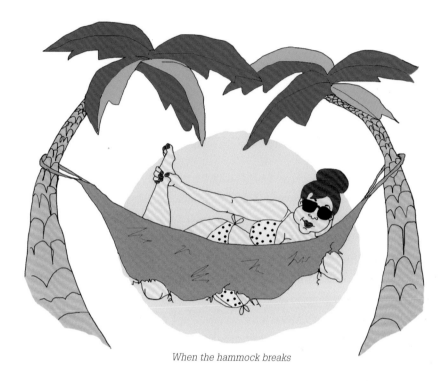

When the hammock breaks

The pelvic floor throws up many barriers to exercise. Lots of women put off asking for help and advice because, let's face it, it can be embarrassing talking about your nether regions. Leaky bladders and bowels, prolapses and pelvic floor muscles aren't easy topics of conversation. They're important ones though, for all women, even if you don't think you have a problem. Read on to find out how to improve and future-proof your pelvic health.

What is the pelvic floor?

The pelvic floor is basically a sling of muscles which supports the organs in your pelvis.

Think of it like a hammock, made of long strands of wool. At the front the hammock is tied to your pubic bone and at the back it's attached to your coccyx (sitting bone). On top of the hammock sits your bladder, uterus and bowel. When the hammock strings are nice and tight, everything is well supported and the organs can bounce gently up and down without any issues. If a heavy weight sits on the hammock it will bulge and some

of the strands of wool break, overstretch
or weaken. Holes then start appearing
and parts of the bladder, uterus or
bowel might start descending through
the gaps.

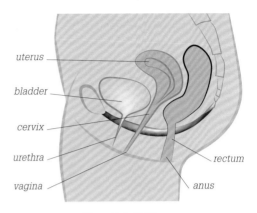

The pelvic floor

What can weaken our pelvic floor?

Anything that adds extra weight or force
to your pelvic floor can weaken it. The
pressure of a growing baby during
pregnancy and the very forceful
contractions of labour are obvious examples. A big baby can often mean more damage
and so can a long, difficult labour or the use of forceps. Not all women who go through a
vaginal delivery will develop weak pelvic muscles but the more babies you have, the
more likely it is. Having a Caesarean section doesn't exclude you from pelvic floor
weakness either. Being overweight, constantly coughing or frequently straining on the
toilet with constipation can all damage the pelvic muscles. Unfortunately, getting older
leaves you more susceptible to problems too. Oestrogen helps to keep tissues supple
and elastic and the further beyond the menopause you are, the less oestrogen there is
circulating round your body. Pelvic floor weakness therefore might catch up with you
later in life, so it's vital to take action before problems arise.

How does a weak pelvic floor affect you?

The symptoms depend upon which part of the floor is weakened and whether there are
any organs bulging through. Let's look at some of the effects of a weak pelvic floor and
see what steps we can take to deal with these problems.

STRESS INCONTINENCE

Activities such as laughing, running, jumping, coughing and sneezing all increase the
pressure inside your pelvis. If the pelvic floor is weak at the point where it supports your
bladder, any sudden increase in pressure can cause urine to leak out. It can be a dribble
or a whole bladder-full. This is called stress incontinence and it affects millions of
women of all ages but as many as half of over-50s. It's a major reason lots of women are
afraid to exercise, especially vigorously. Leaking urine is assumed to be normal after
childbirth, or as you age. Well ladies, this is not true! It's not just 'one of those things'
and if it's happening to you then please read on to see what you can do.

Things to try for stress incontinence

The most important thing you can do is to strengthen your pelvic floor muscles. You need to learn how to exercise them properly. Follow the instructions in the pelvic floor exercises (PFEs) section later in this chapter very carefully. Losing weight to bring you into the normal range

YOU DON'T HAVE TO PUT UP WITH URINE-SOAKED CLOTHES AFTER LAUGHING OR RUNNING FOR THE BUS. TAKE ACTION.

helps stop leaks too. The next step is to see your GP for a referral to a women's health physiotherapist. They'll assess your pelvic muscles and check that you're performing PFEs correctly. Doing regular, good-quality PFEs is the most effective way of reducing stress incontinence.

There are a myriad of products available, both over the counter and online, to help with strengthening the pelvic floor. Many women are spending lots of money seeking a solution. Taking the advice of a specially trained physio will ensure you have the basics right and you can discuss whether you need to invest in anything else to help you. Let's look at some of the devices that are available:

◎ **Vaginal exercisers.** You can make the muscle contractions during your PFEs more effective by using resistance. Inserted into the vagina, these exercisers push back against the muscle as you squeeze. Used for a few minutes a day whilst lying down with your knees bent up, many women find these devices really beneficial. The PelvicToner is an example of a vaginal exerciser and it's available on an NHS prescription.

◎ **Weighted vaginal cones.** These are plastic cones that are inserted into the vagina and they have a small interchangeable weight hanging from the base of them. Start with the lightest one and gradually increase through to the heavier ones once your vaginal muscles can hold them in place for a few minutes a day.

◎ **Biofeedback.** These devices make sure that you're squeezing the right muscles when doing PFEs. A vaginal probe feeds back information about the strength and duration of your muscle clenching. Be warned: they're expensive, and you can't get away from doing the hard work of PFEs. There are some cheaper feedback products which don't use electrical probes; instead a small indicator wand moves up and down when you squeeze the correct muscles.

◎ **Electrical stimulation.** A probe is inserted into the vagina and the pelvic muscles are forced into action by an electrical current; this can be gradually increased to make the muscles work harder. They're particularly useful if your muscles are very weak and don't contract on their own. However, many women don't like the concept and prefer to focus on working the muscles themselves.

Surgical solutions for stress incontinence For 60 per cent of women, PFEs will cure or improve their incontinence but for those who're still affected, the next step is to consider a surgical procedure. There are several options available including tapes that are inserted to support the bladder, stitches to keep the bladder lifted and the injection of 'bulking agents' to strengthen and thicken the urethra (the tube from the bladder to the outside). You should discuss carefully with your surgeon which would suit you best and ask about the risks and benefits of each. You need to feel confident that you're making the right choice for you. Continence surgery is not normally done until you've completed your family.

See your GP if: you're struggling with stress incontinence and don't think you're doing PFEs correctly ▪ you're confident with PFEs but after three months of doing them regularly there's no improvement in your symptoms.

GENITAL PROLAPSE

If your pelvic floor is very weak, your bladder, womb or bowel can all drop down from their normal positions and bulge through the muscular sling. This is called a prolapse and you might be unaware you have one. Sometimes you can feel an aching or dragging and the sensation of 'something coming down'. This might only happen after a long day on your feet when your muscles are tired and gravity has added to the pressure on your pelvic floor. I often see ladies who feel a lump in their vagina and are worried they have a tumour. Having a prolapse can also make sex uncomfortable or painful.

If your bladder is dropping down, then you might have urinary symptoms. These include not being able to empty your bladder properly, incontinence, urgency to get to the toilet and needing to wee more often. If the bowel is descending, then you might get constipated, struggle to fully empty your bowel or need to rush to the toilet. Leaking faeces (faecal incontinence) is sadly common too. I've lost count of the number of times patients have told me they have to use a finger to help pass their motions or press inside their vagina to let a stool or urine come out. Many women are too embarrassed to seek help but be reassured, your GP will have heard it all before.

When the bladder bulges into the vagina it's called a cystocele. When the uterus descends it's a uterine prolapse, and if the rectum is bulging into the vagina it's a rectocele. Have a look at the diagrams on the following page to see exactly what's happening inside us. The amount the organs prolapse varies between individuals.

Once you can visualise what's going on it's easy to see why a prolapsed bladder affects your ability to wee normally. You can also understand why faeces tend to accumulate in the pouch of bowel that forms and why it's hard to get yourself clean; each time you wipe your bottom you're quite literally 'milking' more stool out of the little pocket. Of course you may have a combination of more than one type of prolapse.

THINGS TO TRY FOR GENITAL PROLAPSE

Good quality PFEs are yet again the key to correcting a mild prolapse, or at least stop it getting worse. You also need to reduce the pressure on your pelvic floor so avoiding heavy lifting and losing excess weight will help. Poo can put a lot of strain on your pelvic floor too; avoiding constipation is critical. Not drinking enough fluid is a major cause of this and you need to make sure you have a healthy diet with lots of fruit and vegetables and, if necessary, speak to your pharmacist for advice about laxatives. One tip if you have a rectocele and are struggling to empty your bowel properly is to increase your fibre intake. Fibre helps to bulk up the stools and this can ensure an easier journey through the bowel and a smoother exit from the anus. Straining on the toilet is bad news, and you might find it easier to go if you sit in more of a squatting position. You could squat on the toilet, but a less precarious alternative is to put your feet on a step or a pile of books and lean forwards a little.

I only realised I had a weak pelvic floor when I discovered, to my horror, that I was unable to bounce on my son's trampoline without wetting myself. I also started to notice that I was leaking when running downhill. I saw a GP and a specialist physio and I started doing pelvic floor exercises religiously. I didn't use an electronic toner, I just worked really hard as I didn't want to have surgery. It took months, but gradually, I felt I was gaining more control and the leaks became less frequent. I've gone from feeling 50 per cent sure I won't wet myself when I run to 99 per cent, and I'm proud of that. Siobhan, age 39, mum of two

Larger prolapses or those that are giving symptoms despite PFEs are going to need some intervention. Pessaries are plastic devices, usually in the shape of a ring that are inserted into the vagina and literally hold everything up. They don't cure a prolapse but they help to control it and are very useful if you don't want to have surgery or have been advised against it, perhaps because you still want to have children or have other medical problems making surgery too risky. Many GPs and nurses are happy to insert them and they can be used long term. There are lots of different shapes and types of pessaries available and if necessary you can be referred to a gynaecologist to advise on and fit the right one for you.

The other option for a permanent solution is to have surgery. You should discuss with your surgeon which of the many different surgical techniques would be best for you. There's a small risk that a prolapse will recur in years to come so it's essential to keep up the PFEs and watch your weight.

See your GP if: you think you may have a prolapse ▪ you're having difficulty with passing urine or stools.

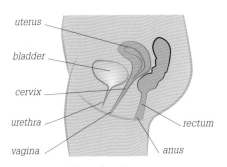

Normal anatomy

uterus
bladder
cervix
urethra
vagina
rectum
anus

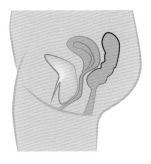

Bladder prolapse

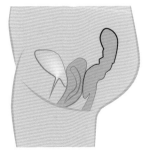

Uterine prolapse

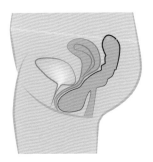

Rectal prolapse

Exercising with a weak pelvic floor

Exercising while suffering with a weak pelvic floor can be a pretty miserable affair. Worrying about wet clothes, discomfort and making the problem worse are just some of the issues to

contend with. Hopefully the advice so far will have spurred you into taking some action but in the meantime there are some other tips that might make staying active just that little bit easier.

Going to the toilet before you exercise is common sense but it's no guarantee that you won't leak or need to go again as soon as you start jumping around. Try the 'double void' technique; this means emptying your bladder twice to ensure it's completely empty. Sit down and have a wee, then count to thirty, put your hands on your knees and lean forwards and see if any more urine comes out. Alternatively, stand up, have a walk about or rotate your hips in a 'hula hula' dance style for a minute and then sit down and try again. Ensuring your bladder is properly emptied can minimise leaks.

Incontinence pads have hugely improved from what they used to be and are much thinner and more discreet. They're still enough to put you off wearing clingy sportswear though. Exercise dresses and skorts (skirts with built in shorts underneath) can be an option to hide any sanitary bulges. A wet pad can cause chafing so applying a barrier cream like Sudocrem can help protect your skin.

It's tempting but not a good idea to limit the amount of fluids you drink before and during exercise. You must stay well hydrated to exercise safely and effectively, particularly in hot weather. If you're heading outdoors for exercise, then planning your route to ensure there's a toilet soon after you start and midway through your journey can give you some reassurance. The Great British Public Toilet Map is a great resource for planning and there are toilet finder apps for toilet location on the move.

There are products on the market that make it possible for you to have a wee while standing up. Small disposable funnels that you position inside your pants which catch the urine and allow you to direct the flow into a bush or a urinal. You'll find women's urinals at large scale sporting events where the portable toilet queues can be excessive. Many women just prefer to squat but it's good to know there are options!

There are some innovative products available to make our exercising lives easier too. EVB Sports shorts were created by a female engineer and are designed to mimic the supporting structure of the pelvic floor. As a result, they can help women with any type of pelvic floor weakness. Clinical trials have shown women feel more confident exercising and leak less urine when they wear them. Don't forget the Diary Doll pants mentioned in Chapter 2; their waterproof panel can protect against small leaks of urine too.

Inserting a normal tampon before you exercise is a trick many women use to give some support and prevent urine leaks. Incostress is a silicon pessary, shaped like a large bumpy tampon. It's designed to stop you leaking urine when you exercise but it also acts as a vaginal exerciser while it's inside to strengthen the pelvic muscles. It can just be popped in for exercise or left in for longer. Have a chat with your GP first to check it's OK for you to try Incostress. It's not suitable if you have a prolapse of your uterus or very weak pelvic muscles.

Urethral plugs are available to buy online. These are basically stoppers that can be inserted into the urethra (the tube which brings urine from the bladder to the outside). You shouldn't use these unless you've been advised to do so by a specialist.

Overactive bladders (OAB)

Many women don't leak urine when they cough, sneeze or run, but they do need to go to the toilet a lot. Their bladders seem to be really small and weak. They live in fear of leaking if they don't make it in time, worry about 'hanging on' during long car journeys and know the location of every toilet in the area. Many spend their days with a pad in their pants or a clean set of clothes in their bag, just in case. They might spend their nights repeatedly getting up for a wee and longing for uninterrupted sleep. This condition is called overactive bladder (OAB) and it affects one in six women in the UK. It occurs at any age but it's more common after the menopause. Urinary leaking associated with this condition is called urge incontinence. It's life-restricting stuff, can make exercising really difficult and we mustn't underestimate the effect it has on everyday life.

THINGS TO TRY FOR OAB

Watch what you drink. Reducing or cutting out caffeine and alcohol can improve OAB. It's tempting to reduce your fluid intake generally, thinking that this will make you need to pass urine less often. In fact, strong concentrated urine will irritate your bladder and make you need to go anyway. If you're exercising hard, fluid restriction is unsafe.

Bladder training. Your bladder will only hold small amounts if you repeatedly empty it, so try to avoid going to the toilet too often. You can retrain your bladder muscle to hold larger amounts of urine by gradually leaving longer and longer between toilet trips. This takes practice and determination; going to the loo every four hours is the target to aim for. Altering your position, changing your activity and distracting yourself can help when you feel the urge to go. It's great if you can track your progress by keeping a bladder diary. For two days write down the times you pass urine and how much you pass (by weeing into a measuring jug), keeping a note of any leaks too. After you've been training your bladder for a few weeks you can repeat this process and see what progress you've made. A bladder diary is a really useful thing to take to the GP if you're going to see them as it gives a really clear idea of the extent of your problems. You can be referred to a continence advisor for help with bladder training.

Medications. If bladder training has been unsuccessful, the next step is a trial of medication to help the bladder muscle to relax. The medications used are from a family of drugs called anticholinergics. They need to be used for at least four weeks to see if there's any improvement. The biggest issue with these medications is their side effects. Often putting up with some minor side effects such as dry mouth, fatigue or constipation is worth it for the improvement you get in your bladder symptoms, but for some they're too intense. Your GP will examine you to check for atrophy (thinning) of your vaginal tissues which is common after the menopause. Using an oestrogen cream in your vagina will replenish and plump up thinned tissues and improve urinary symptoms.

Surgical treatments. Surgery is reserved for very severe cases of OAB and there are a variety of procedures depending on the exact cause and nature of your problems. A technique which is becoming more widely available but not yet fully approved is the injection of botulinum toxin A into the bladder wall to help it relax (yes, bladder botox!). It can be very effective in some women but there's a risk of not being able to empty your bladder properly and the injections do wear off and need repeating.

See your GP if: your overactive bladder is affecting your daily life and you've tried the self-help tips ▪ you notice any blood in your urine ▪ you keep getting urine infections ▪ you feel tired, thirsty or are losing weight and are passing urine more often than normal.

Pelvic Floor Exercises (PFEs)

Learning to do PFEs properly is vital but it isn't easy. It takes time to master the technique and some women find it harder than others. The most important thing to remember is that the exercises need to be done consistently and regularly over a period of months. You wouldn't expect a few bicep curls here and there to make any difference

> **PFEs ARE A VITAL LIFELONG SKILL FOR ALL WOMEN TO HAVE AND WE SHOULD ALL DO THEM REGARDLESS OF WHETHER WE HAVE ANY SYMPTOMS OF PELVIC FLOOR WEAKNESS.**

to your upper arm strength and your pelvic muscles are no different; they need to be trained every day. Once the muscle strength has improved you need to carry on doing them regularly to maintain their power.

HOW TO IDENTIFY THE RIGHT MUSCLES

When you squeeze your pelvic floor muscles no one should know you're doing it. There should be no bottom or thigh movement, no tummy going in and out and no breath-holding or raising of eyebrows! It can be really hard to identify the right muscles, especially if they're weak. Here are four ways to help you find the right ones:

1   **Sit on the toilet for a wee.** When you get midstream, stop and hold your flow of urine for a few seconds. Those are the muscles you want to work. (Don't do this regularly or it might affect the way your bladder empties).
2   **Lie down or sit back on a chair.** Insert one of your fingers into your vagina and try to squeeze your pelvic muscles around it. You might feel a good squeeze, a flicker of movement or nothing at all depending on how strong your muscles are. Try this in a crouching position too.
3   **Pop in a tampon.** Sit on the floor with your knees bent up, lie on the bed, crouch or stand, it's up to you. Pull gently on the tampon string so the tampon just starts to move. Contract your vaginal muscles to try to stop it coming out. You can soak the tampon in some warm water to make it swell a bit if you can't hold it in at all.
4   **Sit on a firm chair with your feet on the ground.** Try to squeeze around your anus like you're trying not to break wind. That's working the muscles at the back of your pelvic floor. Now try to squeeze your vaginal muscles, lifting them as you squeeze. Now see if you can move the squeeze to the muscles around the front of the pelvic floor just as if you're trying to stop mid-wee. Identifying the three areas of the pelvic floor takes practice. It helps if you focus hard and concentrate on the muscle you're trying to work.

HOW TO EXERCISE THE MUSCLES

Once you've identified the muscles it's time to start squeezing them. You can do this anywhere and at any time. Sitting in the car, waiting for the bus and before going to sleep. Combining short squeezes and long squeezes gives the best workout.

- ◎ **Take a breath in.** As you breathe out do five short, sharp squeezes.
- ◎ **Repeat this five times.**
- ◎ **Take a breath in.** As you breathe out squeeze your muscles and hold onto the squeeze trying to lift the muscles at the same time. Think of your pelvic floor as a lift that's slowly going up the levels.
- ◎ **Repeat this five times.** Once you can comfortably do these you can take things up to the next level:
- ◎ **Increase to 10 short sharp squeezes.** Repeat five times.
- ◎ Increase the length of time of the slow squeeze by keeping the squeeze going while you breathe in and out gently and not just for the duration of your outward breath. Make your target 10 seconds of slow squeezing. Repeat five times.

HOW OFTEN SHOULD THE EXERCISES BE DONE AND HOW LONG WILL THEY TAKE TO WORK?

Do these exercises at least three times a day. It'll be four to 12 weeks before you notice any benefit; patience and perseverance are key. You can check for progress by using the 'finger in vagina squeeze'.

PFEs commonly fail because women simply forget to do them regularly. Associate the exercises with something you do frequently like boiling the kettle. Set a reminder on your phone or use an app such as squeezyapp.co.uk. You need to train your brain to remember the right nerve pathways to activate the muscles so consciously engaging a squeeze before you sneeze will eventually lead to it happening automatically.

See your GP if: you can't identify the right muscles to squeeze ▪ there's no improvement in your pelvic floor weakness after 12 weeks of PFEs.

Fanny farts

Vaginal farts, varts or queefs; whatever you call them they don't sound attractive. Air whooshes uncontrollably out of the vagina. They're common during sex but also during floor exercises like sit-ups. Poses in yoga where your legs go above your head literally suck air into your vagina and it's expelled on lowering them. Strengthening your pelvic floor muscles and engaging them before and during these poses might prevent air getting in. Wearing a tampon can help stop them too otherwise it's a case of avoiding certain poses or laughing it off!

Case history

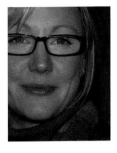

BERNADETTE HOPE, AGE 40, MOTHER OF TWO, HULA-HOOPING
AWAY IN NEW ZEALAND

After the birth of my second child at the age of 32 I decided to
get fit and shed the extra two stone I had hanging around.
Around eight months into my new running hobby I started to get
groin pain; I foolishly continued regardless. One morning when
running to work I felt I needed to go for a poo. I'm a frequent sufferer of constipation and
that morning I felt I'd been carrying a small bowling-ball-like weight on my pelvic floor!

Later that day, as I lifted a heavy box, I suddenly felt a bulge on the back wall of my
vagina and my lower back started to ache. I was devastated; I knew immediately that I'd got
a prolapse. I reluctantly went to see a GP who confirmed that I had a small rectocele and
referred me to a women's health physiotherapist. I was so frustrated that I couldn't run but I
knew it might only make the problem worse.

The answer, although by no means a quick fix, was just good old pelvic floor exercises. I
was guilty of massive neglect of my pelvic floor muscles! I had totally underestimated how
important those muscles are!

I purchased an electronic pelvic floor exerciser and set about my new daily pelvic floor
workout as my toddler had his afternoon nap. My new electronic friend, looking not too
dissimilar to a vibrator, generated raised eyebrows from my husband. Despite my insistence,
he couldn't quite accept that this was hard core pelvic floor training and not just my 'special'
alone time in the bedroom! As the weeks and months passed, my physio confirmed my
pelvic floor strength had greatly increased. I was so proud of myself!

I now run again but also love mountain biking, paddle boating and kayaking. I find body
balance classes and hula-hooping are great for my core strength. I listen to my body and try
never to let a day go by without doing my exercises. I'm now embarrassingly passionate
about pelvic floor health and often have to stop myself bringing up the subject to random
pregnant ladies or runners who pass me! Please don't neglect your well-hidden but
crucial muscles.

Chapter 7

THE MENOPAUSE AND BEYOND

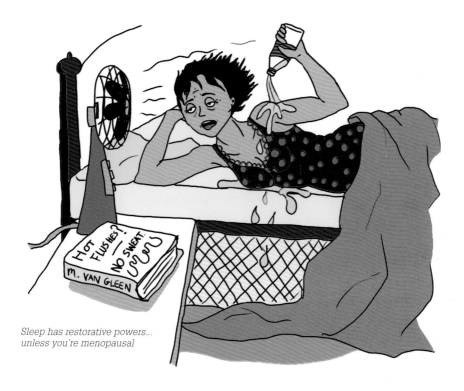

Sleep has restorative powers...
unless you're menopausal

The menopause. The 'change'. The bit when we all get hot, sweaty and grumpy. Some women will be lucky and breeze through it, but for others it's horrendous. You may utterly lose yourself, forget who you are and experience unbearable symptoms for months and, dare I say it, years on end. You may even find yourself at the GP worried that there's something wrong with you. It can be a negative time when women mourn the loss of their fertility and begin to feel old. There are major changes going on in the body and understanding these is the first step in taking control at a time when you often feel powerless. With knowledge and options we can change our perception of the menopause and look on it as a time of new beginnings and opportunities. Let's start talking about it.

What is the menopause?

Before the menopause, your ovaries release an egg (ovulate) every month; this egg has the potential to become fertilised and lead to pregnancy. If fertilisation doesn't happen

It's a weird feeling knowing I'm entering a new era physically and leaving behind certain things. I'll always be a mother and my teenage boys still need me, but I have more freedom on a daily basis to pursue my own interests and time to be outdoors or at the gym. Being 50 is really exciting; there are lots of opportunities ahead and I have a strong network of friends and family to share the ups and downs that I now know are an inevitable part of life. I also feel a quiet personal confidence, that I didn't have in my 30s or 40s, knowing that if I've survived this far (babies, miscarriages, divorce, being a single working mum, losing my mum and helping dad through his cancers) that I have, deep down, the strength to handle whatever life throws at me next. In the meantime, it's about focusing on what and who is important and enjoying the everyday joys of family, friends, love and daily triumphs at work or sport. Looking after yourself in the early stages of menopause is not selfish – it will help you deal with the symptoms, is an investment in your future and you absolutely do deserve it!   Jo from Yorkshire and healthyhappy50.com

then you have a period. When your ovaries stop ovulating and you haven't had a period for 12 months then you've reached the menopause. Your child-bearing years are officially over. In the UK the average age for the menopause is 51. The time leading up to this point is called the peri-menopause. After the menopause women are labelled as post-menopausal. The range of symptoms you can experience around the menopause are mainly due to falling levels of the hormone oestrogen. Hot flushes, night sweats and mood changes are the commonest ones. You can usually expect to have them for about four years but some studies have shown symptoms for as long as 10 years before and 12 years afterwards!

Exercise and the menopause

Exercise can become incredibly difficult around the menopause; who wants to get hot and sweaty in a gym class when that's happening 10 times a day anyway? But exercise can be helpful in managing some of the problems you'll encounter and keeping active is vital for your future health. The Health Survey for England in 2014 showed the number of women who do enough exercise for good health when they're 55 years old is 57 per cent, and it drops down to just 8 per cent by age 85. This is frightening; just because you're getting older doesn't mean you should be less active. In fact the reverse is true: exercise helps to prevent and treat a multitude of medical conditions, many of which are age-related. Exercising through and beyond your menopausal years will:

◎ improve your cardiovascular health, meaning lower blood pressure and reduced risk of heart disease and strokes;

◎ lower your risk of developing type 2 diabetes;

◎ reduce your risk of cancer including breast, bowel and endometrial (womb);

◎ help prevent osteoporosis by maintaining your bone and muscle strength;

◎ help you control weight gain which naturally happens at this time;

◎ reduce menopausal symptoms including mood changes, aches and pains, fatigue and possibly hot flushes;

◎ improve your strength and balance to prevent falls and help you maintain your independence as you age;

◎ lower your risk of dementia.

Bleeding patterns

The peri-menopause can bring heavier, more painful and more frequent periods than you're used to; this comes as a shock to many women. When there's no other medical reason for this it's called dysfunctional uterine bleeding (DUB). It's similar to when your periods first started and your ovaries hadn't quite kicked in to a regular pattern of egg release (ovulation). Periods can become irregular and prolonged too and unexpected bleeds make exercise tricky. Turn back to Chapter 2 for lots of information and tips on how to deal with heavy and irregular periods. One of the most effective ways to manage bleeding in the peri-menopause is an intra-uterine system (IUS). This is a small device which is inserted into the uterus (womb) through the vagina and cervix. It slowly releases a low level of progesterone which over time thins the lining of the uterus and can reduce and even stop periods altogether. This is a fantastic way to make sure that bleeding doesn't prevent you being active. An IUS can stay in for five years and as well as providing contraception it can become part of an HRT prescription if and when you want or need it.

See your GP if: you have bleeding after sex ▪ you're bleeding in between your periods ▪ your bleeding is heavy, irregular and causing you concern ▪ you've had no periods for 12 months and you start having any vaginal bleeding, no matter how small the amount.

Hot flushes and night sweats

Eighty per cent of women will experience hot flushes when they're peri- and post-menopausal. You might just get the occasional flush and night sweat or your life might become intolerable with numerous hot flushes in the day and sleepless nights waking, shivering with sweat-soaked sheets. We call these vasomotor symptoms, and they're your body's way of trying to regulate its temperature.

The distress these symptoms can cause shouldn't be underestimated. Hormone replacement therapy (HRT) can be used as a treatment for sweats and flushes if they're causing disruption to daily life. Have a look at the section on HRT later in this chapter for more information.

Many women prefer to use a 'natural' product to cope with their menopausal flushes and sweats. Unfortunately, the news isn't good. Although there'll always be some women who feel they do benefit from natural supplements, on a larger scale there is, so far, insubstantial evidence to fully recommend them.

Black cohosh is the most commonly used preparation. This is a member of the buttercup family and was traditionally used by Native Americans for a wide range of medical problems. The most recent guidelines from the National Institute for Health and Care Excellence were written in November 2015. They advise that although there's some evidence that black cohosh may relieve vasomotor symptoms, the safety of the many different products available cannot be guaranteed. There's also potential for them to interact with other medications. A Cochrane review (which combines and evaluates multiple medical studies) also found that there's not enough evidence to recommend

I've used running as my main form of exercise for about 15 years. Initially when I hit the menopause my periods stayed regular but became heavy and long. I sometimes flooded through despite super tampons, and there weren't many days that I wasn't bleeding. It made me feel a bit woozy and lightheaded. But, apart from the inconvenience of carrying spare tampons around, and having to make pit stops on long runs, this didn't affect my training. Now, it's quite a different story. My periods are much lighter but my runs are a struggle. I feel like I'm dragging someone else's body along, and it doesn't want to go. It's hard to motivate myself to get out so I've changed to a walk-run routine. I'm not giving up, as I want to look after myself and I'm determined to complete my next marathon.   Karen Stylianides, 52, three marathons and counting...

black cohosh for the treatment of menopausal symptoms. They do, however, point out that many of the studies were of low quality and that further research is needed.

Phytoestrogens are chemicals found in plants that mimic the actions of the female hormone oestrogen and another Cochrane review in 2013 looked at whether they were helpful in reducing hot flushes. Phytoestrogens can be found in foods like soy and alfalfa and in plants like red clover. The idea of a 'natural oestrogen' to top up our falling levels is an appealing one. The review looked at 43 different studies and found that there wasn't any conclusive evidence to prove that taking phytoestrogens would reduce the frequency or severity of sweats and flushes. They highlighted that more studies needed to be carried out on some soy-derived chemicals. There was, reassuringly, no evidence that any of these products would be harmful if used for a short time.

Sometimes doctors prescribe medications other than HRT for vasomotor symptoms. These include the antidepressant medications called SSRIs (selective serotonin reuptake inhibitors) and venlafaxine, which is an SNRI (serotonin and noradrenaline re-uptake inhibitor). Other options are gabapentin, commonly used as a painkiller or to control epilepsy, and clonidine, which is traditionally used to lower blood pressure. All four of these were not designed for, but have been found to have the side effect of, reducing flushes and sweats in some women. If there's a reason you can't take HRT, you have other medical conditions such as depression which might also benefit from taking one of these medications or if other steps to control your flushes have failed then talk to your GP about whether one of these options might be suitable for you.

EXERCISE AND HOT FLUSHES

So far there's not enough evidence to prove whether exercise reduces flushes and sweats. A recent study at Liverpool John Moore's University has shown some promising results, though. A group of menopausal women were asked to improve their fitness through exercise over a period of four months. For comparison, another group of women were asked to just carry on with their normal lives. The lead author of the study, Dr Helen Jones, told me, 'The women who improved their fitness reduced the number of flushes they had by 62 per cent and the intensity of any flushes they did have was reduced by two-thirds. We measured the amount of sweating and skin reddening during a flush and this was significantly less after the exercise training. We therefore

Tips for exercising with hot flushes

◎ Adapt to the weather; exercise outside when the air is cool or in an air conditioned studio on hot days.

◎ Keep well hydrated; sips of ice-cold water are best.

◎ Choose breathable clothes; several thin layers make it easy to cool down or warm up.

◎ Have a cold water spray handy to use on your face.

◎ Avoid caffeine, alcohol and smoking, which can make flushes worse.

◎ Opt for a warm rather than hot shower after exercise.

believe becoming fitter helps your body to become more efficient at regulating its temperature. This was a small study and we're hoping to carry out a larger one to explore this further. If exercise can offer a significant reduction in hot flushes, then many women would choose to improve their fitness rather than take HRT.'

Don't forget there's a link between obesity and more severe sweats; layers of fat provide insulation making it harder for your body to lose heat. Using exercise and diet to help get to and maintain a healthy weight can therefore help. Flushes can also be triggered by stress and exercise is a great way to ease this.

Fatigue

It's no wonder women complain of feeling tired all the time in the peri-menopause with night sweats, trips to the toilet or simply an unexplained inability to sleep. Sometimes you'll sleep well but just feel unrefreshed. There are lots of tips on sleep in Chapter 11. Fatigue, however, can occasionally be due to an underlying medical problem; hypothyroidism is common at this time of life and anaemia can be caused by heavy peri-menopausal periods. Turn to Chapter 11 for more information.

Mood changes

Menopausal mood changes can range from the same irritability you associate with pre-menstrual syndrome through to severe depression. The hormonal changes going on in your body are partly to blame for this but it can also be your reaction to the symptoms you're experiencing and the way you feel about yourself. Coming to terms with the fact your child-bearing years are drawing to an end and realising that your body is ageing can be things women struggle with. We're all different and how you react to these changes is a very personal thing. It's not unusual to feel forgetful, anxious

I decided to join Portsmouth Triathletes club when I was 47. I was absolutely awful at the swimming part so I started swimming lessons. Three lessons in, I had a panic attack and a flashback to nearly drowning when I was a child. I couldn't breathe, couldn't see and was clinging to the side of the pool. Later my mum explained I had nearly drowned and needed to be resuscitated after a friend's mum had let me get out of my depth when I couldn't swim. Anyway, I kept working on learning to swim properly and getting better at it and my instructor made me work harder, which brought on hot flushes! However, hot flushes in water are so much better than hot flushes while running or cycling. In the water there's this cool flow of fluid all around your body and face and neck, and although you do get hot, it isn't so overwhelming. For some reason in water I don't get the palpitations that normally accompany my hot flushes on land although I know I'm working just as hard. One issue I've had is that my skin has become greasier with the menopause so nose clips just slide off. I've had to learn how to swim without one which has been another challenge for me! Dee Kirkby, author

and also angry. You might find it difficult to concentrate too. Being prepared for these feelings and accepting that many are normal can help you cope. You're more likely to suffer from depression around the menopause if you've had post-natal depression or depression linked to pre-menstrual syndrome. Rather than battling on you should seek help. Have a look at Chapter 8 for advice about depression.

Exercise is a really useful tool to help with mood changes around the menopause. We know that exercising causes the release of our body's own happy hormones. It can help to ease stress, anxiety and mild to moderate depression. It can also provide some much-needed laughter with friends or, conversely, quiet time for peace and reflection. Don't underestimate its power to help you mentally at this time of your life. If your motivation is low, there are lots of tips and tricks that will help you. Turn to Chapter 17 for some strategies.

HRT can be used to improve mood changes that are associated with the menopause. If your doctor feels you're depressed, then antidepressants might be needed instead of or in addition to HRT.

See your GP if: you think you might be depressed or you're struggling to manage your moods.

Joint and muscle pains

Aching joints and muscles aren't something you immediately associate with the menopause but they're common. It's usually the neck and shoulders that are affected but it might be your wrists, hips, knees or ankles. It can be difficult to decide what the exact cause of your aches might be because pains from osteoarthritis can be very similar. Osteoarthritis is a type of arthritis that's more common as you age. Have a look at Chapter 12 for more information about it. The good news is that exercise will be beneficial whatever the cause of the pains. Choosing something of low intensity with less impact on your joints is a good option for particularly sore days. A gentle swim, walk or cycle can be effective pain relief. A soak in a warm bath and some simple painkillers like paracetamol or ibuprofen will help too. Deciding to grin and bear the pain and avoiding activity will only make things worse. It's far better to try some exercise and pain relief and get your joints and muscles moving. Remember that the time it takes to recover from exercise will increase a little as you get older. It's important to allow rest and recovery days after hard exercise to allow your muscles, bone and joints to adapt to the stress the activity has put on them.

See your GP if: you have any swelling of your joints ▪ your joint or muscle pains

One of my biggest challenges over the last two years has been waking up early. I started waking at 4.30am and was simply unable to get back to sleep. Nothing worked. It was really affecting my attitude and ability to cope with being a single working mum. I was tearful, stressed and lacking in confidence. I started indoor rowing when a friend suggested it might help me sleep. I'd not been to a gym for literally decades! Within a couple of weeks, I found I was sleeping again and gradually got closer to 6am. I still have bad nights every so often but exercise in the day is a huge help. I just feel better, calmer, stronger, happier and more confident. I've rowed a million metres and a marathon to raise money for Macmillan Cancer Support and after my mum's death from lymphoma in December 2013 I rowed from Edinburgh to Paris over eight months (in a gym!). I didn't expect it to have such an impact on my life as a whole. I fell back in love with being active, grew in confidence and broadened my horizons hugely. It was the best way to enter my 50s and I will always love that crazy rowing machine for the lessons I learned night after night! Jo Moseley, indoor rower, outdoor swimmer, mum of teens

Forgetfulness

Forgetfulness and memory loss are common symptoms of the menopause but they can make you worry that you're developing dementia. If you're concerned about the severity of your symptoms, see your GP to discuss it. We know that exercising regularly is protective against dementia and can reduce your risk of developing it by 20 to 30 per cent. This can be a great motivational drive, especially if you have a family history of dementia or have seen a loved one suffer the devastating effects of the disease.

are not controlled by gentle exercise and simple pain killers ▪ you have joint pain and a family history of rheumatoid arthritis.

Palpitations

Hot flushes and night sweats are often accompanied by a racing heart and a pounding in your chest. We call these sensations palpitations and it's not unusual to feel them during the menopause either with or without a sweat. Turn to Chapter 15 to learn how to deal with palpitations.

Headaches

Really bad headaches can start in the peri-menopause. If you've previously had headaches linked to your periods, then the irregular and often more frequent bleeding around the menopause can result in an increase in headaches. Sleep deprivation is also a trigger and there's plenty of that going on! For those who get migraines, the peri-menopause can be tricky: 40 per cent of women find their migraines are worse. HRT is safe to use if you have migraines and it might help improve them; for others, it can make them worse. It's worth trying HRT that is absorbed through the skin such as a patch or a gel as the level of hormones in the blood is more constant, which is generally better for migraine sufferers. The news isn't all bad, as about 30 per cent of women don't find their migraines are affected by the menopause and 15 per cent find they improve. When you're post-menopausal, hormonal headaches will eventually stop. Headaches triggered by other factors, however, may continue. Turn to Chapter 15 to learn more about headaches.

Vaginal dryness

Oestrogen helps to keep the skin of your genital area nice and moist and bouncy. This acts as a great defence against germs and it also means there's enough lubrication for sex. As oestrogen levels fall when you're peri- and post-menopausal, the skin in this area can become dry, thinned (atrophic) and uncomfortable. This can make sex or even having a cervical smear test painful as the skin of the vagina is less elastic and it hurts to stretch it. Exercise like walking, running or horse riding can cause friction which may irritate an already delicate area, sometimes leading to pain, itching or small amounts of bleeding. This atrophy of the tissues also reduces the skin's ability to keep germs away and that's one of the reasons that many women start to suffer with recurrent bouts of bladder infections around the menopause.

A simple solution is to buy a vaginal moisturiser from the pharmacist. Used regularly or just applied when needed it can relieve dryness. To really solve the problem, you need to replenish the oestrogen in the vulval and vaginal tissues and this can be done using creams, pessaries (tablets that are inserted into the vagina) and flexible rings which stay in place in the vagina; these all contain oestrogen. These need to be prescribed by a doctor who will usually want to examine you first to check there's no other reason for your discomfort. They can all be used long-term and are suitable for the majority of women. If you're already taking another form of HRT but still have vaginal symptoms then these can be used alongside.

Libido

Although many women enjoy a healthy sex life through the menopause, a plummet in sex drive (libido) is common. Vaginal dryness can put you off sex and a lack of sleep or poor self-image don't exactly make you want to spring into the bedroom. Treating the night sweats and vaginal dryness can help. A lack of interest in sex can also be a symptom of depression, which, if treated, can improve your sexual desire. Communication is key: discussing with your partner how you're feeling is vital. Exercise has been shown to improve libido in some studies, although these weren't specifically involving menopausal women. What's clear is that exercise brings a sense of wellbeing and the psychological and physical benefits it provides are undoubtedly going to have a positive impact on your sex life.

Weight gain

Controlling your weight can be a balancing act throughout your life, but never more so than when you hit your menopausal years. You might've been able to lose a few pounds by simply cutting out some treats and doing a bit more walking in your younger years but all of a sudden weight seems to become impossible to shift. It can be frustrating and upsetting and lots of you tell me it's one of the worst things about this phase of life.

Breasts and the menopause

Breasts can change quite significantly after the menopause. The number and size of breast lobules reduces and the skin becomes less elastic. This means breasts might shrink, sag and take on a more 'empty' appearance. It's therefore a vital time to be taking extra care of your breasts with supportive bras, particularly when exercising. Your risk of breast cancer also increases as you get older so you should generally keep an eye on them and report any changes to your GP. Don't forget that exercising regularly can reduce your risk of breast cancer by up to 20 per cent. See Chapter 3 for more information.

Weight seems to pile on around your middle and it's easy to get demoralised and end up in a spiral of weight gain. This will have a significant impact on your future health so you need to be pro-active in finding a solution that works for you.

WHY DO WE GAIN WEIGHT?

It'd be nice if weight gain was simply down to falling oestrogen levels and topping them up would solve the problem. Unsurprisingly it's not quite as simple as that and, as always, it's different for each of us.

The way your body deals with food intake changes; it switches into storage mode. A larger percentage of your consumed calories are converted and stored as fat. The energy your body needs to function and to just keep ticking over is called the Basal Metabolic Rate (BMR). As you get older your BMR decreases and therefore so does your requirement for calories. If you keep on eating the same amount, you'll gradually put on weight. One of the things affecting your BMR is the amount of muscle in your body – your muscle mass. Muscle mass steadily declines after the age of about thirty, a process called sarcopenia; it's part of ageing and happens to everyone, even the most active. Sarcopenia becomes more pronounced after age 50. Muscle uses lots of energy (calories) to function and when there's less muscle our BMR is reduced and fewer calories are required to fuel it.

You'll also gain weight if you move less. Although you might not think women move less at this time of their lives the statistics tell us differently. The Health Survey for England 2009 Trend Tables shows that activity decreases with age and by age 75 only one in 20 women are active enough for good health. Subtle changes in lifestyle might account for this. Many women find they get more time for themselves when they aren't constantly meeting the demands of small children. As a consequence, it's easy for sedentary time to increase. There's an assumption that you should slow down as you age; activities on offer seem to be more sedate and less intensive. The opposite should be true; you should be increasing your activity and moving more.

If your mood drops during the menopause you might find yourself comfort-eating and drinking more alcohol. Getting motivated to exercise and eat healthily can be a struggle. Life can be stressful at any age but when relatives are ageing and work and other family issues combine, stress levels can be particularly high. Sleep disturbance and chronic tiredness pre-disposes you to stress. Your levels of cortisol and other hormones increase with stress and if they're high for long periods of time they can affect the way energy is used and stored in the body and cause weight gain.

All these factors make it easy to understand why women tend to gain weight around the menopause. It's important to mention that there's no clear evidence that hormone replacement therapy (HRT) causes weight gain. It's just used at a time when the natural tendency is to gain weight. It can actually help some women lose weight by improving sleep, mood and motivation.

RISKS OF WEIGHT GAIN

The problem with weight gain around the menopause is that the fat tends to settle around your middle. This is called central obesity and means there's a higher chance of fat being stored around our internal organs (visceral fat). See Chapter 1 for more on the dangers of visceral fat. The risk of getting most diseases like heart disease, diabetes, cancer and dementia, increases with age. If your background risk is rising and you allow extra risk from enlarging visceral fat stores, you're asking for trouble.

WHAT CAN YOU DO ABOUT WEIGHT GAIN?

So far the picture is looking bleak but there are solutions! First, you need to approach the whole issue with the right attitude. You need to make positive changes in your everyday life. If you do nothing, then the natural course of events is that you'll gain weight. If you're already active, you'll have to make some adjustments to what you do.

It takes a lot of discipline to keep my weight under control; it's a constant battle nowadays. Excess weight impacts on my quality of life and I know it adds to any age-related health problems. To stay healthy requires constant self-denial, something that can get very boring. How do I keep the motivation and discipline going? Donna Champion, age 53

Specialist opinion

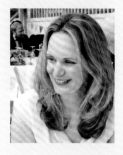

DR HANNAH SHORT, GP WITH SPECIAL INTEREST IN WOMEN'S HEALTH AND THE MENOPAUSE. LOVES TEA AND TRAVEL

HORMONE REPLACEMENT THERAPY (HRT)

The use of HRT remains a controversial topic. Years ago it was touted as the answer to all our aging ills and doctors prescribed it with gusto. However, since 2002, prescriptions for HRT have plummeted. This followed the publication of the results of two large-scale studies: the Women's Health Initiative (WHI) and the Million Women Study (MWS). Serious concerns were raised over the safety of HRT, particularly in the area of heart disease and breast cancer.

The validity of both studies has since been called into question and we can now be reassured by the publication of the National Institute for Health and Care Excellence (NICE) Guidelines on Menopause in November 2015. All the evidence has been weighed up and we're advised that for most women, if started within 10 years of the menopause, the benefits of HRT will largely outweigh the risks. It should only be taken for as long as is necessary at the lowest effective dose. Importantly, we can be happy that many of the risks associated with HRT do not apply to women under the age of 50 years. Moreover, women who are diagnosed with Primary Ovarian Insufficiency (POI), and those who have an early menopause (under 45 years of age), should be encouraged to use HRT up to the natural age of menopause in order to reduce the risk of osteoporosis and heart disease.

HRT can be a very effective way of treating hot flushes, aching joints, palpitations and mood swings. It can be taken as a tablet, applied to the skin (as a patch or gel), placed under the skin as an implant (not widely available in the UK) or inserted into the vagina as a cream, pessary or ring. You can expect to start feeling better within four weeks and see the full benefits at around three months. The route you opt for will depend on your past medical history and your lifestyle; for example, if you swim daily, a patch or gel are probably best avoided. Conversely, if you suffer with migraines, you may actually be more suited to a patch because it offers a more even delivery of hormones.

The type of HRT you need will depend on where you are in the menopausal timeline and whether or not you've had a hysterectomy. Continuous oestrogen-only HRT is given to women who've had a total hysterectomy, but if you still have a womb, progestogen (manufactured progesterone) is also an essential component to reduce the risk of womb cancer. Your doctor can discuss your different options.

Don't suffer in silence.

Understanding why you gain weight makes it easier to prevent it.

◎ **Eat well.** Look honestly at your diet. If you include all your sneaky snacks and glasses of wine, you're probably not eating as healthily as you think. I'm not suggesting you cut out all treats and pleasures but your body's requirements are changing.

◎ **Reduce sedentary time.** Minimising how long you spend sitting makes a big difference. If long hours at the computer are unavoidable then take short movement breaks every half an hour. Plan walks with friends rather than sitting down for a coffee. Walk instead of getting the bus. You get the gist; moving little and often is the key.

◎ **Build muscle.** Combat sarcopenia by preserving and increasing your muscle mass. Adding in two 30-minute sessions of weights to your weekly routine means you'll gain muscle, which uses up extra calories and helps prevent central weight gain.

◎ **Increase time and intensity.** What if you're already doing plenty of exercise but the weight's still going on? Sometimes you need to mix it up a bit; try something new or put in extra effort. Working out for longer or just working harder can help. For example, if you swim twice a week and do 50 lengths then why not try to swim every fifth length as fast as you can? It's easy to sneak in a bit of extra effort in everything you do.

Bone health

Bone mass, bone density, osteopenia, osteoporosis, fragility fractures: it can all sound very confusing. Bone health isn't actually a complicated topic and it's one we all need to be aware of. There are many positive steps you can take to look after your bones and being well-informed can have a significant impact on your wellbeing in your later years.

BACK TO BASICS

Adults have 206 bones in their body. Bones are an amazing piece of engineering because they're incredibly strong but also very light. Far from the pale inert shell you might picture, they're actually a hive of activity and very much alive.

In the centre of bone there's a hollow cavity filled with a jelly-like substance called bone marrow. Some of the marrow is yellow and is a fatty tissue and the rest is red bone marrow where blood cells are made. Some bones such as the femur (thigh bone), pelvic bones and ribs have lots of red marrow and produce large quantities of blood cells.

Around the marrow is cancellous bone; it looks spongy but it's still strong. Compact bone is what we think of when we picture bones: smooth and hard, it surrounds the softer cancellous bone. The periosteum is a thin layer covering the surface of all bones, containing nerves and blood vessels which branch into the bone, bringing nourishment.

Bone is not a static structure. It's being destroyed and reformed all the time. Cells called osteoclasts are continuously breaking down bone to release minerals like calcium (which is used for blood clotting and nerve pathways) and other substances such as growth factors that are stored inside. While the osteoclasts are munching up bone there are osteoblasts working alongside them to form and replace the bony tissue. It's a never-ending cycle ensuring bones release their goodness but remain strong too. It also means that if a bone is injured there's a process in place that will quickly heal the damaged area.

BONE STRENGTH

Bone grows rapidly throughout childhood, the osteoblasts are working harder than the osteoclasts and more bone is being made than broken down. By age 18 you have 90 per cent of your bone mass. It peaks when you're about 30 years old; this is when your bones are at their thickest and strongest. After this age you lose slightly more bone than you gain. When you reach the menopause there's a sudden surge in bone loss for a few years followed by a slower, more steady decline over many years.

How can we measure bone strength? Your bone density (also called bone mineral density or BMD) gives an indication of your bone strength and can be measured in a variety of ways. The most common uses a special X-ray technique called a DEXA scan. DEXA stands for Duel Energy X-ray Absorptiometry and it measures how many of the X-rays fired at the body are absorbed by the minerals, such as calcium, in the bones. The more that are absorbed, the denser the bone. The density of the hips and spine are the most commonly measured and the results compare your bone density to that of a 30-year-old woman, to give an idea of your risk of future bone fracture.

Before you all rush off to try and book yourselves a DEXA scan, remember, not every woman needs one, particularly if you're under 50 years old. You need a discussion with your nurse or GP to determine your fracture risk and decide whether a scan is needed. They might use a computerised calculation called a FRAX™ score to help make the decision.

If any of the following apply to you, you should ask for a chat about your fracture risk:

◎ You're over 65 years old.

◎ You've had an early menopause (before you were 45 years old) and haven't taken any HRT. This may be a natural menopause or by having your ovaries surgically removed.

◎ You've fractured a bone when you've only had a minor injury (we call this a fragility fracture).

◎ You have to take steroid tablets for more than a total of three months a year for a medical condition.

◎ You're over 50 years old and underweight, with a BMI of less than 19.

◎ You're over 50 years old and smoke or regularly drink more than 14 units of alcohol a week.

◎ You're over 50 years old and your parents have osteoporosis or have had a hip fracture.

◎ You have other conditions that affect bones, such as rheumatoid arthritis.

◎ You aren't menopausal but haven't had a period for a year.

◎ You have a condition that affects how nutrients are absorbed into your gut, such as coeliac disease or inflammatory bowel diseases like Crohn's disease.

OSTEOPENIA AND OSTEOPOROSIS

If your bones are starting to show signs of 'thinning' it's called osteopenia. Once bone density reaches a certain low point, bone strength is significantly reduced and you have osteoporosis. The osteoblasts can't keep up with the bone destruction by the osteoclasts and your bones are weaker, more fragile and at high risk of fracturing (breaking). The most common bones to break are the wrist, hips and vertebrae (spine bones). It might not take very much impact at all to break an osteoporotic bone and even a minor fall can result in a fracture; we call these 'fragility fractures'. There are nearly 9 million fractures in the world every year caused by osteoporosis and fragility fractures are estimated to cost the UK £2 billion a year. The consequences of a fracture can be huge. Wrist fractures can cause problems with the use of your hands, hip fractures need major surgery to fix and vertebral (spinal) fractures can mean long-term pain. This is why it's so important to do what you can to preserve your bone health.

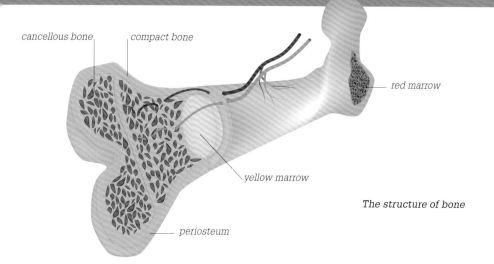

cancellous bone compact bone

red marrow

yellow marrow

The structure of bone

periosteum

What can you do to preserve your bone health? If you have osteoporosis, then your doctor will discuss drug treatments with you. These aim to slow down the activity of the osteoclasts and boost the osteoblasts to try to maintain or even improve bone strength. A healthy lifestyle will help protect your bones at every age but if you've been diagnosed with osteopenia or osteoporosis then make sure you're doing everything you can to improve your bone health.

Here are some top tips:

◎ Stop smoking. Smoking slows down the osteoblasts which are trying to make new bone.

◎ Reduce your alcohol. Stick to the current guidelines of no more than two units of alcohol each day.

◎ Eat a healthy balanced diet. Check the diet tips on the next page for advice.

◎ Get outside. Vitamin D is vital for strong bones and exposure to sunlight can provide this. In the autumn and winter (or throughout the year if you usually cover your skin) consider taking a 10 microgram vitamin D supplement daily to ensure an adequate supply.

◎ Exercise regularly. This is crucial for preserving and improving bone health. Read on for advice about the best types of exercise to do.

EXERCISING FOR HEALTHY BONES

Although 90 per cent of your bone mass is established by the age of 18, it's never too late to start exercising. Weight-bearing exercise is great for bones; anything that involves standing on your feet or making some impact with the ground counts. It might be a high-impact exercise like running, skipping, dancing or a sport that involves

Specialist opinion

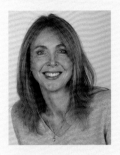

KATE PERCY; COOK, MUM OF THREE, SERIAL MARATHON RUNNER
AND AUTHOR OF GO FASTER FOOD AND GO FASTER FOOD FOR KIDS
WWW.GOFASTERFOOD.COM

EATING AS WE AGE

It's an unfortunate truth that as we age we can no longer get away with eating just what we fancy! It's not all doom and gloom though. Incorporating careful food choices into an active lifestyle can serve as damage limitation. First, make every calorie count! Nutrient-rich foods such as wholegrains, pulses, starchy fruit and vegetables, lean meat, eggs and fish will help you feel fuller for longer, sustain energy and boost your immune system while preventing the pounds from piling on. Be totally honest with yourself, especially with 'empty-calorie' refined sugars and foods high in fat. Do you really need that second glass of wine, slice of cake or that Frappuccino?

Eating within 30 minutes of your workout will speed up your recovery as well as reduce your susceptibility to fatigue, joint and muscle damage. The following foods, in particular, may help you keep active for longer:

◎ Milk and natural yoghurt. Rich in bone-strengthening vitamin D, phosphorus, potassium, calcium and magnesium to prevent stress fractures and osteoporosis. Other great sources of calcium are cabbage, broccoli and kale, pulses, nuts, dried fruit and sardines (eaten with bones).

◎ Kiwi fruit, pomegranates and blueberries. Antioxidant-rich foods such as these can build protection against damaging free radicals and even slow down the ageing process, as well as promote muscle repair, minimise muscle soreness and stiffness and help boost the immune system.

◎ Almonds. Just a small handful of almonds gives us a surprisingly hefty contribution towards our recommended daily allowance of important nutrients to help promote strong bones, healthy teeth, skin and hair, favourable blood cholesterol levels and to protect against cardiovascular disease and even cancer. Particularly efficient at regulating blood sugar levels and sustaining energy levels, almonds are packed with vitamin E, B vitamins and protein, plus healthy, mono-unsaturated fats and minerals such as calcium, iron, magnesium, phosphorous and zinc.

jumping, such as netball or gymnastics. Lower-impact exercises such as walking, low intensity aerobics or simple stair-climbing are beneficial too. Anything that gives your body a bit of a jolt as you do it will stimulate bone formation.

Non-weight-bearing exercises like swimming and cycling won't specifically improve bone strength but can form part of your general exercise routine to improve your fitness.

> WEIGHT-BEARING EXERCISE, MUSCLE-STRENGTHENING AND BALANCE ACTIVITIES WILL ALL HELP TO PRESERVE YOUR BONE HEALTH AND REDUCE YOUR RISK OF FRACTURE.

It's now known that muscle-strengthening exercises are also an effective way to strengthen bones. Muscles are anchored to bones by tendons and when a muscle is used the tendon tugs on the bone and stimulates bone thickening. You need to keep gradually increasing the weights that you use to get the most benefit. You may not like the idea of weight training but it's important to know it's excellent for bone health. Ideally we should do it two or three times a week with a day off in between sessions.

EXERCISING WITH OSTEOPOROSIS

It's normal to feel nervous about exercising if you have osteoporosis. There's no simple answer as to what's safe; it depends on how severe your bone thinning is, which bones are affected and what activity you want to do. You should discuss your personal risks with your doctor. The National Osteoporosis Society provides some brilliant resources to help you decide what activity is right for you and how to look after your bones. This includes a helpline where you can discuss your condition with a specialist nurse.

Menopause and cardiovascular health

The risk of cardiovascular diseases such as heart disease and strokes increases as you age, particularly after the menopause. High blood pressure, diabetes, high cholesterol, smoking, obesity and a family history of cardiovascular disease all increase your risk too. You can't change your genetics but it's great news that exercising regularly will help control all of the other risk factors and reduce your risk of heart disease and stroke by up to 30 per cent. It can even help smokers quit. You can discuss your risk of cardiovascular disease with your GP and if you're seeing them about the menopause this is an ideal time to raise the issue.

Case history

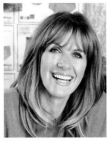

CAROL SMILLIE – TV PRESENTER AND DIRECTOR OF
WWW.DIARYDOLL.COM

It always makes me laugh when people assume that because I'm slim, I'm therefore fit. The reality is that I loathe exercise, and have spent most of my life avoiding it like the plague.

Now that I'm 54, and in the menopause, the changes in my body have been both fascinating and unwelcome.

My most shocking moment came on holiday, as we met up with friends for a dinner in the local beach bar. What could be nicer than the sun setting, guitar music and an evening of great food and company?

As I stood up to welcome them, I felt my insides literally fall out. I've never been so grateful to be wearing black leather jeans and my DiaryDolls, but as I ran across the beach bar to the toilet, I found the Ladies' was occupied, so I had to use the Gents'. Like a scene from Texas Chainsaw Massacre, there was blood everywhere. I scraped together what little loo roll there was, and returned to my seat, ashen-faced. My darling husband, quietly passed me napkins under the table, and covered for my forced bonhomie, for which I was eternally grateful. It only happened once, but I now have the utmost respect for those women who experience heavy bleeding regularly.

In general, my mood is generally pretty calm (a lot better than when I had periods, my husband reliably informs me), my hot flushes are not unbearable thus far, as I've always been the coldest woman alive, but the thickening of my waist and legs is utterly depressing. My pelvic floor needs some attention too, as a third sneeze is always a worry.

I've launched myself on a 10-week programme with a hypnotherapist and holistic women's specialist to see if small changes can make a difference. I have flax seeds in smoothies, Epsom salts in my bath, a protein- and plant-based diet and yes, a little gentle exercise, including pelvic floor routines at the traffic lights when I'm driving. Rome wasn't built in a day, but I'm definitely getting there.

It's all a balancing act of benefit versus risk. If you've already had a fragility fracture or are felt to be at high risk, it makes sense to avoid activities that are high impact or where you're likely to fall. This means sports like skiing, football and horse riding aren't suitable. The problem comes, however, when you're really proficient at an activity, you love it and don't want to give it up. You might feel your personal risk is low. That's when a discussion with your doctor can help you to decide what's right for you.

THE RISKS AND BENEFITS OF A PARTICULAR ACTIVITY ARE DIFFERENT FOR EVERY ONE OF US AND SHOULD BE ASSESSED ON AN INDIVIDUAL BASIS.

As a general rule you should avoid high-impact activities like running, jumping and exercises that put stress on your spine like sit-ups and lifting while bending and twisting. Low-impact activities like walking, dancing and climbing stairs are perfect. Cross-trainers provide great low impact exercise. Weight lifting to strengthen muscles should ideally be done, under the supervision of a trained instructor. Exercise that improves balance and co-ordination is fantastic for preventing falling and broken bones. Yoga is ideal but take advice from an instructor about which poses are safe. Why not try something new like Tai Chi?

My GP wasn't happy with my weight; I've always been on the light side. She referred me for a bone scan and I was devastated when the scan confirmed low bone density in my spine. I went into meltdown for a while. At this point I'd been running for about nine months and I decided that I would keep going but be sensible. I don't enjoy weight training but I've found some routines that suit me and I know it will strengthen my muscles and bones and stop me getting injured. I'm terrified of frosty, icy or snowy days in case I fall and break something. Inspired by my children, I decided to take up karate. I'd read that karate is a good thing for people with osteoporosis to learn as it's great for balance and teaching you to fall safely. My instructor is aware of my condition and makes sure I do it safely. If you're diagnosed with osteoporosis, don't be afraid to get out and exercise. It's really important for your mental and physical health. Get one or two walking poles for the winter for stability and confidence if you're out and about on an icy day. Sinead Bradbeer, 44, experimental baker

Chapter 8

MENTAL HEALTH

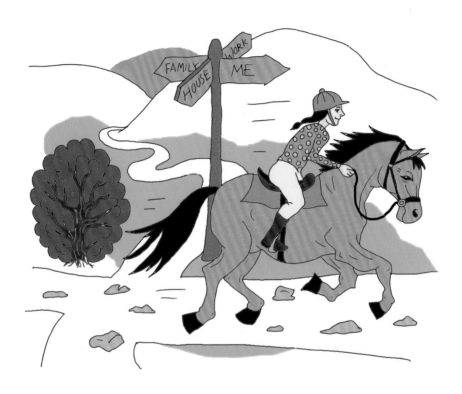

Why is it so acceptable for people to seek advice when they feel unwell with an infection but not when they have a problem with their mood or feelings? Both make you unable to carry out your daily lives, both make you vulnerable and in need of support. Somehow, sadly, mental ill health is often seen as a sign of weakness. No one likes to feel weak or unable to cope and many women battle on for months pretending that everything is OK and hoping that their feelings will just go away. This is very isolating, which only adds to the problem. Mental health problems have nothing to do with your intelligence or resilience. There's no need to feel guilt or shame; things go wrong mentally in the same way as they do physically. It can happen to anyone; yes, all of us are at risk of mental illness.

What's going on in our brains?

Many parts of the brain are involved in regulating your mood and emotions and the most important ones are collectively called the limbic system. The limbic system communicates with the areas of brain around it via nerve cells (neurons)

which use chemical messages and electrical impulses to relay information. There are an estimated 90 billion neurons in your brain.

Neurons don't actually touch each other and the small gap between them is called

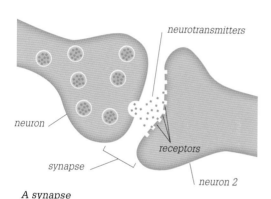

A synapse

a synapse. Electrical impulses can't cross a synapse so the information is turned into a chemical message for this part of the journey. These chemical messages are called neurotransmitters and they transfer information across the synapse to receptors on the neighbouring neuron. It's a clever system because only certain neurotransmitters will fit the receptors on the other side. Think of it like a children's shape sorter toy; if the shape fits correctly in the hole, the message will go through. The speed at which this happens is staggeringly fast; just think how quickly you move your hand when you touch something very hot.

So, how does this translate to your mental health? Well, you might have heard the names of some neurotransmitters; serotonin, dopamine, and noradrenaline. Having too much or too little of a transmitter, or receptors that don't work properly, will upset the transfer of messages around your brain. The communication between the different parts of the limbic system therefore gets disrupted, which affects your response to situations, your emotional stability and memory pathways.

Other important chemical messengers are hormones. Your endocrine (hormonal) system is responsible for the production and balance of these. Different glands around your body produce hormones, ranging from oestrogen released by your ovaries to cortisol from your adrenal glands (near your kidneys), which is released in response to

> LOTS OF SMALL STRESSORS ADD UP. YOU CAN'T DO EVERYTHING. DELEGATION AND ASKING FOR HELP ARE GREAT SKILLS TO LEARN.

stress. The brain acts as the control centre, monitoring hormone levels and adjusting production where necessary to try to keep everything in balance. Your endocrine and nervous systems are closely entwined. It's easy to understand how a small message error can affect the balance of the whole complex system.

Common mental health problems

It's normal to feel a variety of ups and downs, particularly when life gets difficult and you're thrown into emotional or stressful situations. At what point you feel you have a mental health problem can be difficult to determine and will certainly be different for each of us. No one fits neatly into diagnostic boxes and the point at which women ask for help varies hugely. Let's consider some of the most common problems and see how they affect you. Have a look at the self-help section for tips to help all of these conditions and read how exercise can act as therapy for them too.

STRESS

Stress is a common and major problem in society today. The Health and Safety Executive reported that in 2014–2015, work-related stress accounted for 43 per cent of days off work in Great Britain. That's a huge and worrying figure. What causes stress to one of us may be a walk in the park to another; we're all different. Your coping skills also vary day to day according to what else is going on, such as how much sleep you've had or where you are in your menstrual cycle. Whatever your situation, anything that puts a demand on you has the ability to cause stress.

Stress can leave you feeling overwhelmed, inadequate and unable to think straight.

I started skiing when I was 28, because my then boyfriend (now husband) was a mad keen skier. I was totally rubbish in my first week, but I just loved the sense of being out in the mountains. Crisp, clean cold air, gorgeous views and nothing to think about except what my body is doing at that time. My mind is totally empty when I ski, I am completely in the moment. So as well as being amazingly good physical exercise, skiing is a great benefit to my mental health. Jo Sacks, 43, GP, ex ski holiday rep and marathon runner

It's draining and exhausting yet often you can't switch off or sleep because of the constant churning of thoughts in your mind.

See your GP if: you've tried the self-help measures and are still feeling overwhelmed ▪ you have physical symptoms but don't know what's causing them.

ANXIETY

It's entirely normal to feel anxious about important events and many of us are worriers by nature. Sometimes, however, this turns into more than simple overthinking. Anxiety can happen to even the most laidback of us. About one in 20 of us are struggling with symptoms of anxiety right now and it's more common in women than men.

When you're anxious you have high levels of stress hormones and neurotransmitters. These include adrenalin and cortisol which are released when you're in a dangerous situation. This is called your 'fight or flight' reaction, it's your body's emergency mode which is activated if your survival is at risk. Breathing and heart-rate increase and you feel hyper alert. When you suffer with anxiety, your brain starts seeing normal things as threatening, triggering your emergency mode inappropriately. It's exhausting! Sudden feelings of nervousness over simple tasks, irrational fears about ordinary situations and a general sense of not being fully in control can be overwhelming and scary. Anxiety often focuses around one particular issue such as health, constant worrying that there's something seriously wrong with you or your loved ones, but more often it's a general anxiety about everything and nothing. It can be disabling and restrictive and stop you being able to function normally.

Physical symptoms as a result of mental strain

Genuine physical symptoms can be triggered by your emotional state. It's your body's way of telling you it's under pressure and needs some help. If you're stressed or anxious you might sweat, shake or feel your heart racing. Nausea, headaches and changes in appetite or bowel habit are also common. If you're constantly tense you can get pains in your abdomen, chest, neck and across your shoulders. This wide range of symptoms can lead to worry that there's something else going on. If you're in doubt, check with your GP but be reassured that if they suggest it's related to your mental health, it doesn't mean they think you're making it up, just that the solution lies in addressing your mental health problems.

You might have a panic attack; your breathing suddenly quickens, your pulse races and you have a sensation that something really bad is about to happen. It can quickly spiral out of control leading to hyperventilating (over-breathing), shaking or even passing out. You can then live in fear of having another panic attack as they're so unpleasant. They can start out of the blue and catch you by surprise or they can be predictable, building gradually when you're exposed to a situation that makes you feel anxious.

Anxiety often makes it hard to leave the house and it's easy to become reclusive, preferring the safety of your own four walls. It's common to start thinking that everyone is looking at you and judging you and you can become very self-conscious. It can be hard for others to understand why you can't even complete a simple task like going to the shops.

See your GP if: you're suffering frequent panic attacks ▪ your symptoms of anxiety are affecting your everyday life ▪ you're losing weight, have shaky hands (a tremor) or frequent palpitations ▪ you aren't making progress with the self-help tips.

I have a very active imagination and a brain that often charges off further and faster than the rest of me can keep up with. This has led me into a number of periods of stress when I've been keen to impress or contribute to an exciting piece of work, which at its worst included full-on panic attacks. I've learned a lot about many different ways to help myself including diet, mindfulness and time away from social media, but exercise has been my single biggest help. I now run or cycle before work most days. My state of mind when I reach my desk in the morning is clear and well-paced. I make better decisions about balancing my time so I don't take on too much. I can't overstate how much this is down to exercise.   Claire, 30, civil servant, singer and runner

I used to hide away from life due to suffering with anxiety and panic attacks. Since taking up regular exercise my anxiety has almost gone; if it does reappear at any point then a good gym session or a run will keep it at bay again. The accomplishment of doing it, especially when I didn't feel like it, is very rewarding.   Charly, 40, accountant

DEPRESSION

Depression is a poorly understood condition with lots of taboos surrounding it. It can happen to all of us, regardless of which rollercoaster of life we're on. If it happens in response to a bad situation like a bereavement or period of intense stress, we call it reactive depression. It can also come without an obvious trigger and this is called endogenous depression which means 'from within'. Endogenous depression can be very confusing and patients often say to me, 'I don't understand, Doctor, I've nothing to be depressed about.' Even if you don't experience depression yourself, understanding it can make you more effective at helping any of your friends and family who do.

Everyone's experience of depression is different but these are some of the symptoms you may have:

◎ feeling sad, crying a lot and becoming emotional over small things;

◎ difficulty concentrating on a task and being forgetful;

◎ hating yourself and losing your self-esteem;

◎ doubting yourself, lacking self-confidence and finding it hard to make decisions;

◎ disrupted sleep, including not being able to get to sleep, frequent waking and waking up early in the morning. Also sleeping a lot;

◎ excessive tiredness;

◎ feeling restless, agitated and impatient;

◎ thinking, moving or speaking more slowly than usual;

◎ poor appetite or over-eating.

I've had depression and anxiety from the age of 18 triggered by a difficult life of abuse, domestic violence and bad relationships. I think I blame my past on myself. I wonder why it happened to me and what I did to deserve it. I've never had any self-confidence whatsoever. I overthink and worry all the time. My paranoia, jealousy and low self-worth made all my relationships fail; I couldn't trust anyone. Ever since I started going to the gym and eating more healthily I've noticed a huge difference. I'm so much happier. I have more energy and look forward to and appreciate every day. I love going to our local forest with my kids and the dog. If the kids have stressed me out, just going for a quick walk around the block clears my head and I feel like a new woman! Paige, mum of two boys, trainee make-up artist, lover of coffee with friends and junk TV

> IF YOU HAVE DEPRESSION YOU CAN'T JUST 'PULL YOURSELF TOGETHER'. RECOVERY TAKES TIME, PATIENCE AND SUPPORT FROM OTHERS.

◎ not getting any pleasure from the things you would normally enjoy doing;

◎ feeling antisocial and avoiding contact with people;

◎ a lack of interest in sex;

◎ feeling overwhelmed and unable to see a way forward;

◎ thoughts of wanting to run away from everything;

◎ thoughts of wanting to hurt or harm yourself in some way;

◎ thoughts that it would be better for everyone if you were dead and considering how you might end your life;

◎ strange experiences like hearing voices, seeing things that aren't really there or sensing that someone or something is watching you, controlling you or influencing you in some way.

You won't experience all of these and the degree to which they affect you depends on the severity of your depression. It's normal to feel some of these from time to time. Feelings of sadness, poor concentration and self-doubt are part of the normal spectrum of feelings, but if you find that these are happening every day for more than two weeks, aren't getting better and are interfering with your normal life then you should start to consider if you might be depressed and seek help.

See your GP if: you think you're depressed ▪ you aren't making any progress despite trying the self-help steps ▪ you have any thoughts or feelings about harming yourself, ending your life or are experiencing any of the 'strange experiences' listed above ▪ your depression is affecting the way you're caring for your children or carrying out your job.

SELF-HELP FOR MENTAL-HEALTH PROBLEMS

◎ **Recognise.** The first and biggest hurdle is to recognise and admit to yourself that there is a problem. Don't beat yourself up; this isn't your fault, you're not to blame for feeling the way you do. Once you can accept this it's easier to ask for help.

◎ **Share.** Pretending that you're OK and putting on a brave face all the time is exhausting. Constantly making excuses for yourself is not helpful or productive.

Sharing how you feel with someone is very therapeutic and will immediately help to lift the burden. Let them help.

◎ **Get informed.** The more you understand about your condition, the easier it is to accept it isn't a weakness and find ways to control it. There's a list of great places to go for information in the 'Useful websites' section at the back of this book.

◎ **Get back to basics.** Go back to the basics of eating well, maximising sleep and exercising; these often get forgotten when you're struggling. Don't look at the big picture, it's too overwhelming – focus on the now, the next few minutes, hours or days, whichever you can cope with. Avoid using alcohol, caffeine or nicotine as a coping mechanism.

◎ **Relax.** It's essential to regularly schedule time for yourself. Whether you're stressed, anxious or depressed, you need to allow your mind time to switch off. Choose something you enjoy doing that will distract you, whether it be soaking in a bath, watching a film or going for a swim. Have a look at the 'mental wellbeing action plan' later in this chapter for more ideas.

The turning point for me was about three years ago. It was the day I thought I was going to die. It was only when I happened to catch my reflection in the mirror that the impact of what I was about to do hit me. It felt like a sudden kick in the face. I knew something had to change but I couldn't get help, or rather I wouldn't. I'm not sure how I decided that introducing exercise into my life would help; I just remember starting a 30-Day Shred DVD, hoping that what I'd heard about exercise as distracting and endorphin-releasing was actually true. I'm not quite sure what my thought process was. Over the following months I started to notice I could cope better with everyday events. I was beginning to look forward to working out. Looking forward to anything had been absent before. I started to feel less like I was existing in some kind of void. Within a year, I started to look at life and myself in a new way and the only thing I'd changed was to introduce exercise. The positive changes in my body shape reinforced this and it gave me the confidence to seek out new activities. I even joined a running club and became (slightly) more sociable. I definitely became more confident in my ability to overcome barriers, both mental and physical. I've found that exercise has been paramount in changing my outlook. Although the depression still exists, it no longer controls me.
Nicola, 40, academic, weight lifter, runner and occasional obstacle racer

I've been a long-term sufferer of depression. Unfortunately, mental illness seems to run in the family, with both my mum and dad being affected. I struggled with medication in my 20s, it did nothing for me, and counselling seemed to exacerbate things. When I started running it gave me a new focus in my life, something positive to achieve. Targets of a single mile quickly built up to complete races. Soon I couldn't do without running. It gave me drive and confidence and made me feel amazing. Over the course of two years I went from non-runner to running my first marathon and losing four and a half stone in weight. If I don't run I feel bad but the second I get out there and feel the wind in my hair, the mud splattering my legs and hear the birds in the trees, I feel alright and at peace with the world.   Helen, 37, school receptionist

◎ **Take small steps.** Setting yourself small daily targets will help to build your confidence and self-esteem. It's vital that the target is something you can realistically achieve so you succeed rather than fail. It may be something as simple as putting on a load of washing or making a phone call.

◎ **Use resources.** There are lots of resources available to help, from books to online CBT (cognitive behavioural therapy). Counselling services, such as the Samaritans, are available by phone too. Apps like 'Headspace' help with relaxation and anxiety management. There are more ideas in the 'Useful websites' section at the back of this book.

◎ **Be patient.** Recovering from mental health problems takes time, a lot of time. It's normal to have bad days, everybody gets them. Don't focus on them, just accept them, try to get through them and look forward to a better day ahead. Try not to get frustrated with yourself and focus on one day at a time. You will get better.

Exercise and mental health

When you exercise something wonderful happens! Your body releases chemicals called endorphins. These are neurotransmitters, often referred to as 'opiate-like' because they have a similar effect on the body to opiates, a group of drugs which include morphine. Opiates and endorphins bind to the same receptors, producing a feeling of happiness and reducing pain levels. Laughing, sex and good food also cause endorphin release and we know how good these things make us feel. It's fantastic to have this free supply of feel-good chemicals available to use.

With a big release of endorphins, you might experience a feeling of ecstasy or euphoria. You've all heard the phrase 'runner's high', and we know that with prolonged or intense exercise like running it's possible to experience an overwhelming sense of positivity and wellbeing. This doesn't happen every time and many runners haven't experienced it. In all my years of running I've only had two episodes of what I would call a true 'runner's high'. One was in the final mile of the Liverpool half marathon and the other was at mile 21 in my second London Marathon. These stand out for me as I recall feeling like I was floating, all pain disappeared and I began calling out to the runners around me, shouting encouragement and feeling that I was invincible. Surreal experiences indeed, but they demonstrated to me the power that endorphins have on mind and body.

EXERCISE AS THERAPY

Exercise can be used not only to prevent mental health problems but to treat them too.

- ◎ **Exercise makes you feel good.** The release of endorphins during exercise and for a number of hours afterwards lifts your mood in the same way that antidepressant medications do. One of the most common groups of antidepressants is the selective serotonin re-uptake inhibitors (SSRIs) that include medications like fluoxetine, citalopram and sertraline. SSRIs increase the amount of the neurotransmitter serotonin. When there's more serotonin in the synapses, there's a higher chance of receptors being activated and happy messages being passed around the brain. Exercise isn't a replacement for drug therapy for everyone, but it's an important part of a treatment plan.

- ◎ **Exercise calms you.** It can either make you forget about your worries for a short while or allow you time to think and problem-solve. The rhythmic thud of feet on the pavement, the spinning of the bike wheels or the gentle splash of the water on the pool side provides a meditative atmosphere. Often what seemed a major stressor before you set off seems a small hurdle you can jump over when you get back.

- ◎ **Exercise builds confidence.** Stress, anxiety and depression can all knock your confidence and exercise can help to re-build it. Setting and completing little targets and challenges makes you feel good and you'll grow in confidence. Working towards a goal also helps you to look forward more positively; have a look at the 'Goal setting' section in Chapter 17.

- ◎ **Exercise helps sleep.** Nights tossing and turning are common with mental-health problems. Exercise during the day will make sure you're physically tired which helps you get a good night's sleep. Some people find vigorous exercise just before bed is too stimulating but do experiment as this doesn't affect

> MANY WOMEN HAVE DISCOVERED THE POWER OF EXERCISE IN MAINTAINING THEIR MENTAL HEALTH AND WONDER HOW THEY EVER GOT THROUGH LIFE WITHOUT IT.

everyone. Gentle exercise like walking or stretching can help you unwind in the evening.

◎ **Exercise brings support.** It's tempting to want to shut yourself away when you feel low but exercising with others is a very powerful tool. Team sports are perfect for helping you feel included and valued. It can take a lot of courage to sign up and turn up but finding a team where you feel welcomed can give you a sense of belonging which helps your confidence. Any exercise which has a sociable element can help. Gatherings of like-minded individuals opens the door for friendships and the simple act of sharing a hobby is therapeutic. There are many clubs, formal and informal, all over the country, ranging from badminton in the village hall to parkrun (www. parkrun.org.uk) on a Saturday morning. Even arranging to exercise with one friend will give you benefits in terms of motivation and support.

◎ **Exercise is flexible.** Even if you don't feel able to leave the house there are activities you can do. Try exercise DVDs or online classes. Home gym equipment can be picked up cheaply, and what about the good old skipping rope? Half an hour of exercise may feel overwhelming but three blocks of 10 minutes feels much more achievable.

Talking therapies

Talking therapies are powerful for all types of mental-health problems. They include simply having the opportunity to vent your feelings, counselling about specific problems and more advanced behavioural techniques such as cognitive behavioural therapy (CBT) and psychotherapy. A trained professional can equip you with lifelong skills to change the way you think about yourself and your situation. Challenging and emotive, talking therapies require you to speak honestly and openly about your feelings. They're also hard work as there's 'homework' outside of the session and you'll need to practise the techniques. You might have a long wait to access these therapies but remember, these are skills for life.

A mental wellbeing action plan

If your mood is low, you're stressed, tense and just not content with how you feel, take action. Take the calendar and write one of these activities on at least three days in the next week. Plan to do them and make them happen. It may take a lot of willpower but it will remind you that pleasure often comes from simple things.

IF YOU'RE TAKING MEDICATION FOR YOUR MENTAL HEALTH DON'T STOP IT WITHOUT SPEAKING TO YOUR DOCTOR.

- **Go for a walk.** Halfway round just stop and stand still. Concentrate on each of your senses. What can you hear, see, smell, feel and taste?
- **Soak in a deep bubble bath lit by candles.**
- **Arrange to meet a close friend for a coffee.**
- **Do something nice for a stranger;** smile at them or help them with their shopping bags, for example.
- **Watch a really funny film.**
- **Sit, close your eyes and listen to a piece of music you love.**
- **Bake a cake.**
- **Sort out one of the drawers in your house that won't close because it's so full of stuff.**
- **Try a new sport;** dust off that old bike or ask a friend to try a new dance class with you.
- **Ring up or write a letter to someone you haven't spoken to for a long time.**
- **Paint a picture.** Go on, just try – you might surprise yourself.
- **Volunteer for something.** Popping in on an elderly neighbour or helping at a charity event are two suggestions.
- **Learn a new skill.** Look for a course you could do, something you've always fancied, from car maintenance to creative writing, saxophone-playing to pastry-making.

A checklist for mental wellbeing

Every few months it's a good idea to run through a checklist to make sure you're looking after your mental health. When life gets busy it's easy to just pile more and more demands on yourself and leave very little opportunity to take time for the most important thing: you. To be in good shape mentally you need to make sure that different areas of your wellbeing are satisfied and that you feel fulfilled physically, psychologically, spiritually and socially. Here are some questions you should ask

Green exercise

Exercising outdoors surrounded by nature brings extra benefits in terms of mental health. A study carried out by Glasgow University used data from the 2008 Scottish Health Survey to confirm that trees and grass help to calm us down, with woodlands and forests having the biggest stress-busting effect. It can be hard to wander far from home if you're struggling with your mental health but exercise outdoors, such as a walk in a park, is well worth the effort.

yourself, and if you aren't happy with any of your answers warning bells should ring and you should take steps to make changes.

- ◎ Am I doing anything that challenges me?
- ◎ Am I regularly doing anything creative?
- ◎ Have I had a day in the last month when I had nothing planned and just relaxed?
- ◎ When did I last have a good laugh?
- ◎ Am I spending enough time with the people that mean the most to me?
- ◎ Am I constantly feeling overloaded and under pressure?
- ◎ Am I regularly being active doing something I enjoy?
- ◎ When did I last do something to help someone else?

Self-esteem, body image and eating disorders

As a GP, one of the things that strikes me is how close the link is between a woman's view of her body and her mental health. For many of my most depressed patients their weight has been a major factor causing them to feel low in self-esteem and lacking in confidence. Most commonly they've been overweight; any loss of weight has led to a boost in mood and any gain has led to further negative feelings about themselves. This often results in a downward spiral of comfort eating, further weight gains and lower mood. Of course, the opposite is often true; at times of stress and depression many women lose their appetite and weight begins to drop off. If you're underweight you can feel just as self-conscious about your body as those who are overweight.

Over- and under-eating are often a feature of mental-health problems. Over 50 per cent of women with an eating disorder report feeling depressed. It's estimated that over 750,000 people in the UK are affected by eating disorders but it may be much higher than this, as many don't report it to a doctor. The most well-recognised types of eating disorder are bulimia nervosa and anorexia nervosa.

Medication and mental health

It's common to think of medication as a 'last resort' for mental-health problems and something to turn to when nothing else has worked. This only adds to your sense of failure and it's important to understand that medication often has a vital role to play in helping you to get better. It obviously depends on your individual circumstances and the severity and type of your symptoms as to whether or when you should start medication. You need to take advice from a professional. Think back to what's actually happening in the brain: correcting the chemical imbalances is an obvious thing to do. Medication can be crucial in changing the way your brain is working and sits well alongside the other therapies such as talking therapies, self-help and physical activity. If your doctor suggests using medication, see it as a positive step towards getting better rather than a negative one. There are many to choose from and they're too numerous to discuss here but make sure you feel happy with the one you're trying and speak to your doctor about any concerns.

In bulimia nervosa sufferers have a constant pre-occupation with their bodyweight and shape and don't feel in control of their eating. Typically, they binge eat large amounts of food and then feel so guilty that they try to lose the weight they think they've gained from the excess calories. They might do this by vomiting, taking medications such as laxatives to cause diarrhoea or water tablets to dehydrate themselves. Starving themselves or doing excessive amounts of exercise are other common ways to try to shed the perceived weight gain. It's a constant emotional see-saw of gain and loss that can be hard to get off.

Anorexia nervosa is characterised by under-eating due to a fear of becoming fat and a distorted body image where sufferers believe they're much fatter than they actually are. Using methods like self-induced vomiting and over-exercising to prevent weight gain are also common. Weight loss in anorexia nervosa can lead to lots of health problems including feeling tired, cold and constipated. Weight can fall to dangerous levels and infertility, osteoporosis, heart problems and ultimately death can be the result.

It's usually in the late teens that eating disorders strike. A comprehensive survey by the UK charity Beat found that 62 per cent of respondents started developing some features when they were under 16 years old. It's essential that anyone suffering from an eating disorder seeks help. The earlier you ask for help the better, as you're more likely to make a full recovery and there's less chance of your problem becoming recurrent.

Case history

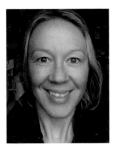

YVIE JOHNSON, 35, MUM OF THREE, TRAINING FOR A 1686-MILE WORLD RECORD ATTEMPT RUN FOR MENTAL HEALTH AWARENESS AND EQUALITY IN SPORT

I've always used sport as a means of keeping me in a place where I can love and challenge myself. I started running aged 23, post-baby number two, in order to be mentally and physically strong for joining the police. Police Sports UK offer lots of opportunities and I threw myself into everything available to make me feel good and boost my confidence. It also gave me a social life that, with children and a demanding job, I didn't really have, and that was essential for my wellbeing. The swimming instructor suggested I train for a triathlon which I'd never even considered. My colleagues told me I was crazy and it would kill me. Their disbelief became a reason to succeed. Within ten months of my first triathlon, I was selected for the Great Britain age group triathlon team. Since then I've done mountain bike duathlons, cyclo-sportives (with Victoria Pendleton), four-day long adventure racing and aquathlons.

I resigned from the police when I had a breakdown and had to be hospitalised. I was diagnosed with bipolar disorder. Exercise has again brought me out of a deep rut; it fires up my confidence like nothing else. It makes me fierce, and determined to stay well. I now use running as a means of losing the weight brought on by my medication, to help get me out of the house and to give my mind a break from the head chatter. I run for peace of mind, not for speed. I've taught myself to focus on the colours, the sounds of birds, the sky and clouds, changing seasons and quirky details that I'd normally miss with my head down. I run with a camera and I blog about my runs to record my thoughts, feelings and images to indulge my creative side. Running is now my way to manage my mental and physical health.

See your GP if: you're struggling to keep a normal eating pattern and think you may have an eating disorder.

Sporting legend Chrissie Wellington spoke openly in her book, *A Life Without Limits*, about her problems with an eating disorder. Here she shares how she has learnt to look at her body in a different way. Let's all try focusing on how amazing our bodies are and what they're capable of.

Case history

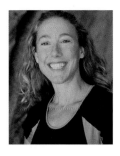

CHRISSIE WELLINGTON, FOUR-TIME IRONMAN TRIATHLON
WORLD CHAMPION, HEAD OF PARTICIPATION FOR PARKRUN
AND MUM TO ESME

The relationship I've had with my body has changed over time, and hasn't always been an easy one. For some of my young adult years I disliked many aspects of my external body. I compared myself, self-depreciatively, to others. I would stand in front of the mirror, my mind full of criticism at the image that stared back at me. I ignored the fact that I had a body that enabled me to achieve the highest academic grades, to play sport, to climb mountains and to live my life to the full. That was around 17 years ago. Today I have a very different relationship with my body. I try not to judge it on its external appearance, but for what it does for me, day in day out. Further, I see my body as a unique combination of my mother and father, and those two people are my shining light – to criticise my body is to criticise them – and that is something I would never do. I have to say I'm moving towards the point where I can say I love my body, inside and out.

My body is what has enabled me to work in jobs I love, to travel all around the world, to participate in a range of sports, to write, to paint, to enjoy music. It's taken me to the top of the world by enabling me to become four-time Ironman Triathlon World Champion and given me the gift of a beautiful daughter.

I push my body and mind to their limits, and even though I haven't always treated my body with the respect it deserves (aside from a few niggles and, recently, a few self-inflicted broken bones) it has never let me down. It heals itself, withstands the pressures I place on it and as such I have come to trust it. It is this faith in my body and mind that's allowed me to reach the huge highs and overcome the lows that come with training and racing. Of course I'm never satisfied, and I continue to strive to get more out of myself and my body, testing it, challenging it and reaching for the stars. I don't look in the mirror and think I'm gorgeous but I'm slowly developing a love for the image that stares back. I'm so grateful for everything my body has enabled me to achieve.

Chapter 9

THE DIGESTIVE SYSTEM

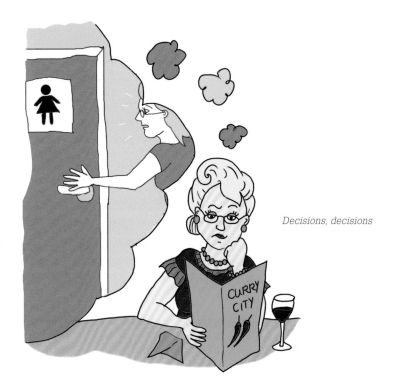

Decisions, decisions

Starting at the mouth and extending right through to the anus, the digestive system or gastrointestinal tract cleverly digests food, extracts the goodness from it and transports the waste to the outside. It's a complicated yet efficient system and for most of us it works with only the occasional hitch. Some of us aren't so lucky and battle daily with problems that can be embarrassing and, if we're honest, a bit gruesome at times. In this chapter we'll look at some of the commonest issues, how they interfere with exercise and, most importantly, what you can do about them.

Biology basics

Let's go back to biology class for a reminder of what the gastrointestinal tract actually looks like.

The journey starts in the mouth, where food is mashed, chewed and squirted with saliva to begin digestion. The muscular oesophagus (gullet) then takes a few seconds to propel food down into the stomach. Here, gastric juices full of acid and enzymes work on the food and it becomes a mushy liquid as the muscular wall of the stomach churns it all about. It's then slowly allowed into the small intestine, which is about seven metres long; food takes around four hours to travel along it. Here, it meets bile which is made in the liver, stored in the gall bladder and squirted into the small intestine to digest the fat in our food. Juices are added from the pancreas which, together with a variety of other enzymes, ensure that fats, protein, carbohydrates, vitamins and minerals are all broken down and absorbed into the bloodstream. The next stop is the large bowel or colon, which is a wider tube than the small intestine. It's about two

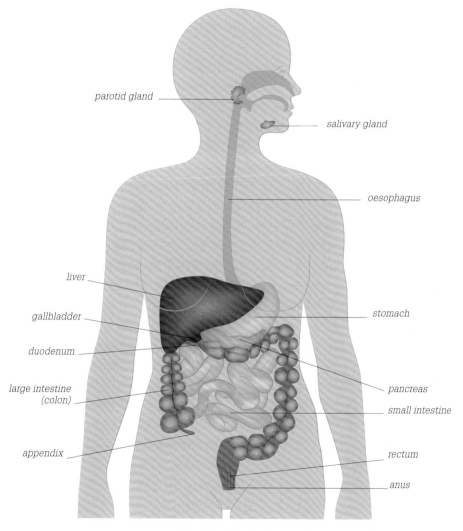

The digestive tract

metres long and it's here that fibre and some starch in your diet is broken down by bacteria that produce gas as a by-product; some of us produce more than others! Water is also reabsorbed in the colon so you end up with a firm stool. This stool sits in the rectum and when this starts to build up and stretch the rectal wall you get that feeling of needing to poo. Thankfully, for most of us the muscles of the anal sphincter only allow that to happen when we're good and ready.

Irritable bowel syndrome

Irritable bowel syndrome (IBS) is incredibly common. It's estimated that up to 20 per cent of people in the UK suffer from it, but it may be much higher than that as there are lots of people who simply cope with the symptoms and don't go and see a doctor. Women are twice as likely to suffer from it as men and it tends to strike when we hit our 20s but it can start at any age. It varies from mildly inconvenient to severely debilitating.

WHAT IS IT?

There's a lot we don't understand about IBS. The bowel seems to simply become over-sensitive, leading to a range of symptoms including abdominal pain, bloating, diarrhoea and constipation. These symptoms may come and go and you might not get all of them. They're usually worse first thing in the morning and after you eat, and opening your bowels often eases them. You might feel that other symptoms in your body link to your IBS, such as back ache, fatigue and urinary symptoms. Sex in certain positions can also be uncomfortable with IBS.

HOW DOES IT INTERFERE WITH EXERCISE?

Exercising when you're bloated and uncomfortable can be really hard. Wearing tight clothing and jumping around isn't appealing. Diarrhoea is common with IBS and it's often accompanied by a sudden and urgent need to go to the toilet. This is frequently worse in the morning and it can take more than an hour and several trips to the toilet for things to calm down enough for you to leave the house. Exercising early in the morning is difficult, and you then have the challenge of fitting it into another part of your day. Sudden urges for the loo can strike at any time and you might not want to go too far from home when your IBS is bad. It can be a real confidence knocker and very limiting. Knowing what to eat and when can be tricky, particularly if you're training for an event and want to use energy drinks, gels or foods which may simply not agree with you.

WHAT CAN YOU DO ABOUT IT?

IBS can be a lifelong condition. It can't be cured but it can be 'managed' and you may have long spells when you're symptom-free. You need to become an expert in your own IBS and explore what works (and doesn't work) for you.

Have a look at the 'tips for troubled tummies' later in this chapter for advice on how to cope with a tricky bowel. Although you might find dietary triggers,

for some women it's just the actual act of eating and activating the gut that brings on IBS symptoms, rather than any specific foods. If diarrhoea is your main problem it might help to reduce your dietary fibre; on the other hand, if you're constipated, increasing fibre can be beneficial. If you're increasing your fibre some studies show you should increase 'soluble fibre', which is found in oats, fruit and root vegetables, rather than 'insoluble fibre' from bran, wholemeal bread and brown rice. However, remember we're all different and experimenting is the key. What you drink plays a role too; caffeine, fizzy drinks, alcohol and fruit juices can make things worse. Managing IBS is always a case of trial and error and just when you think you've got it sussed you have an unexpected flare-up and are left scratching your head again. Trying to keep a well-balanced, healthy diet and minimise bowel symptoms can be a daily challenge.

There's a close link between our emotional state and IBS. We don't fully understand this but stress and tension can lead to a flare-up of symptoms. Talking therapies can be helpful if there's a strong emotional element to your IBS and there's some evidence that hypnotherapy can help ease abdominal pain. Simple relaxation is something you can try at home. Interestingly, some medications used for anxiety and depression help control IBS. The improvements in pain are separate to the mood benefits and help people with IBS who aren't depressed. Low doses of these medications seem to help pain perception and have some direct action on the bowel itself.

A pharmacist is a great resource for advice on which medications you can use to ease bowel spasm, bloating, constipation and diarrhoea. If they feel that a medication on prescription would be more suitable they'll direct you to your GP.

Exercise has an important role to play in managing IBS. It stimulates the bowel, which can ease and prevent constipation. It also acts as a great stress reliever; it's a powerful coping mechanism for you to have up your sleeve. Finding a healthy, productive way to use up nervous energy can make a positive difference to your symptoms.

'Some is better than none' is a good rule to remember. You may not feel up to your usual regime or confident enough to go far from a toilet but there's always something you can do. On a bad day, just exercise at home using a DVD or online class. Even simple stretches while wearing loose clothing is better than nothing.

See your GP if: you're having recurrent abdominal pains or bloating and don't know why ▪ you have frequent constipation, diarrhoea or a mixture of both ▪ you've been told you have IBS but your symptoms aren't controlled or they've changed ▪ you have weight loss, bleeding from your bottom or a family history of bowel or ovarian cancer.

Runner's trots

The sudden need to open your bowels when exercising has been named the 'runner's trots'. It happens in all types of exercise but it's particularly common in runners, causing emergency detours to find toilets or crouch in hedgerows. It can happen even if you aren't normally affected by bowel troubles such as IBS. The exact mechanism isn't known but it seems to be a combination of things that causes it.

Exercise causes a surge of adrenalin which is helpful for increasing your pulse and heart rate, but also speeds up bowel emptying. 'Pooing your pants' with excitement and fear happens at any age! When the stool moves quickly through the bowel there's less time for liquid to be reabsorbed making it watery and explosive. Pre-race nerves can cause fluttery tummies and an annoying urge to go and empty your bowels; that's adrenalin in action.

I've had IBS for 10 years now so I'm well used to it but it still occasionally infuriates me. Despite being very careful with my diet I do get flare-ups which can impact my lifestyle considerably, stopping me from working or exercising due to painful cramps. I row for my university and I've had to adapt my food in ways my crew mates don't have to. My coaches recommend sports drinks in order to refuel and sugary sweets before long head races; my crew mates use them but they give me bad cramping and diarrhoea. I have to make sure my breakfast gives me the fuel I need for races, even though I won't be racing for a couple of hours. I used to try to eat nearer to the time of exercise; this made me feel more energetic while racing but it led to a pretty unpleasant situation post-exercise! Despite altering my eating for it, I do think exercising has helped my IBS due to the stress relief it provides. Mary, 20, university student and rower

As you run your bowel jiggles around, which irritates it and makes it want to expel its contents. Added to this, the bowel needs a good blood supply to work normally but when you're exercising, your muscles take priority, so blood is diverted away from your bowel, affecting its function.

If you have weak pelvic-floor muscles, the pressure that the lower loops of bowel places on your pelvic floor when you run can be too great and you simply can't hold the stool in. Turn to Chapter 6 for advice on how to solve this.

Using concentrated sports gels and drinks can upset some tummies, especially excessive consumption of them over long distances. Not everyone gets the runner's trots but for some the inconvenience and embarrassment can be a real barrier to exercise. Have a look at the 'tips for troubled tummies' for ways to overcome this.

Tips for troubled tummies

It's really a game of trial and error because we're all different and what works for one of us might not work for another, but here are some things to try if your exercise keeps being interrupted by tummy pains, diarrhoea or wind:

◎ **Eat slowly.** Chew food properly and don't eat on the move.
◎ **Time your eating.** Leave plenty of time for digestion before exercise; two to three hours for a meal and an hour for a snack.
◎ **Choose food wisely.** Watch out for 'trigger foods', they may be rich, spicy or too fibrous. Keep a food diary to identify the culprits, and remember it may be what you ate the day before that counts.
◎ **Avoid caffeine.** It improves alertness and performance but it stimulates the gut. Some sports supplements contain caffeine, so check the label.

My IBS started shortly after the birth of my first child. I have symptoms, to a greater or lesser degree, every day. For me, the biggest thing is needing to go to the toilet when I run. There are some days when I know it isn't worth even attempting it. I'm careful what I eat beforehand, especially if I'm training for a half marathon or running in a race. I always wait two hours after breakfast and make sure I go to the toilet (preferably two or three times!) before I run. I know where the public toilets are on all my routes; there are four on the eight-mile route I use for half marathon training! Sarah, mum of three and keen runner

- **Try eating 'normal food' during endurance sports.** Bananas, bagels, dates and homemade energy bars, for example.
- **Step up training slowly.** Suddenly increasing time, distance or intensity can upset the bowel. It's better to make steady, gradual changes.
- **Relax.** Stress and tension only add to tummy problems. Stay calm before an important event with relaxing music, imagery, distraction and deep breathing.
- **Hydrate well.** Bouts of diarrhoea cause significant losses of fluid and body salts so keep hydrated with fluids containing electrolytes.
- **Consider medications.** If nothing else helps, it's safe to use an anti-diarrhoea tablet like loperamide. Be aware that side effects include cramps and constipation.
- **Be prepared.** Plan a route to include toilet stops and pack tissues in your pocket.
- **Practice makes perfect.** For an important event, stick with tried-and-tested methods and don't experiment.

Coeliac disease

We used to think that coeliac disease only started in childhood and was responsible for children with diarrhoea who just didn't thrive or grow properly. We now know that this is only a very small part of the whole picture and the one in 100 people with known coeliac disease are probably just the tip of the iceberg.

WHAT IS IT?

Coeliac disease is not a wheat intolerance or an allergy; it's one of the many autoimmune conditions where, for an unknown reason, the body starts to produce antibodies to attack itself. In coeliac disease the body becomes sensitive to the protein gluten that is found in wheat, rye and barley, resulting in damage to the lining of the bowel. The normal lining of the small intestine is disrupted and this leads to diarrhoea,

I tried lots of different strategies in terms of timing or types of food stuff, and all to no avail. It was worse when I was going faster; slow jogs weren't a problem and neither were cycling, rowing or swimming. I had a bit of an issue in races so I always ran in dark pants! I did end up planning routes around public loos and favourite bushes; I just got used to carrying tissues and going with nature! I was underweight but funnily enough, since I got myself back to a healthy weight it doesn't seem to be a problem. Annabeth, runner, artist and yoga lover

Inflammatory bowel disease – IBD

Inflammatory bowel disease (IBD) is entirely different to irritable bowel syndrome (IBS). The most common types of IBD are Crohn's disease and ulcerative colitis. The lining of the gut wall becomes inflamed and unable to function properly, leading to diarrhoea, mucous or blood in the stools and abdominal pains. These are lifelong conditions that can't be cured, only managed. Many women with IBD have mild symptoms and only the occasional flare-up that doesn't require any treatment. Others have resistant symptoms requiring specialist input, nutritional supplements, medications and possible surgery to remove the sections of inflamed bowel. IBD usually starts in your late teens and early 20s, but it can happen at any age. While exercise won't prevent IBD, it can help ease the stress of coping with a long-term condition and can also help prevent osteoporosis, which is more common with IBD.

bloating and abdominal pain, but also to fatigue, weight loss and insufficient absorption of essential nutrients. Poor nutrient absorption leads to health conditions such as anaemia and osteoporosis. Untreated coeliac disease can also affect fertility, and sufferers are more likely to have problems in pregnancy.

HOW DOES IT INTERFERE WITH EXERCISE?

There's no reason why anyone with coeliac disease can't exercise normally and even perform at the highest level. It generally causes more problems if you remain undiagnosed and are struggling with symptoms of pain, diarrhoea, fatigue and poor nutrition. After diagnosis, if you follow a gluten-free diet you should start to feel much better and find that your energy levels and exercise tolerance return to normal. There's still a risk of poor absorption of certain nutrients including iron, vitamin B12 and folate, which can all result in anaemia. Anaemia causes tiredness; you might need a blood test to rule this out if you're struggling. If diagnosis has taken some time or your coeliac disease is poorly controlled, your bones are at risk of osteoporosis. Have a look at Chapter 7 for advice and information on osteoporosis.

There are plenty of gluten-free foods that will fuel you for exercise. Most sports drinks and supplements don't contain gluten, but it's always worth checking the labels before trying anything new.

Having coeliac disease increases your risk of certain rare types of bowel cancer. Following a gluten-free diet will, over time, reduce this risk back to almost that of the general population.

WHAT CAN YOU DO ABOUT IT?

Doctors routinely check for coeliac disease if patients complain of bowel symptoms or fatigue. A positive blood test means coeliac disease is likely, but for proof you need to be referred to a specialist to have a biopsy of your small bowel. The results might be inaccurate if you've already switched to a gluten-free diet. The current advice is to eat some gluten in more than one meal a day for at least six weeks before the test.

Once diagnosed, you should follow a gluten-free diet, even if you don't have any symptoms; there are lots of resources to help such as the charity Coeliac UK. Some gluten-free foods are available on prescription in the UK. It's useful to see a dietician when you're first diagnosed, if you're having problems with your diet or your symptoms aren't settling. An annual check with your GP will make sure you're not developing any of the complications of coeliac disease.

See your GP if: you think you have coeliac disease ▪ you have a strong family history of coeliac disease ▪ you have coeliac disease but your symptoms aren't well-controlled.

Acid reflux

Gastro-oesophageal reflux or GORD is the medical name for what most people call heartburn or acid reflux. There's a tight muscular valve at the lower end of the oesophagus called the oesophageal sphincter. This sphincter closes to keep down the watery, acidic contents of your stomach. If it doesn't close properly, juices track back up

I'd been running for a year or so before I was diagnosed with coeliac disease. When I went gluten-free I noticed I had much more energy and felt lighter mentally as well as physically. The fact that I no longer had to worry about whether I'd have to cut short a run to get to a loo was a weight off my mind. I also noticed that the headaches that had plagued me on a weekly basis stopped, which meant I could run more frequently. The other benefit of running, for me, as a post-menopausal coeliac, is that it helps improve bone density and wards off the threat of osteoporosis.   Helen, 58, teacher (reflux) into the oesophagus. This gives a burning feeling behind the breast bone. You might also get nausea, a cough, a sore throat, pain when swallowing and bad breath. It's a common condition, particularly if you're overweight, pregnant or have a poor diet. You might only get it occasionally after eating, especially if you've overindulged, but it can be a frequent, if not daily, problem which, if left untreated, can cause inflammation of the oesophagus, ulcers and in rare cases oesophageal cancer.

HOW DOES IT INTERFERE WITH EXERCISE?

Reflux can be worse after eating and when lying down. Exercising too soon after eating will make you feel sick and cause heartburn. This is particularly true for floor-based exercises when you lie flat or stretches and yoga poses when you're in the head-down position. Sometimes you can literally feel the acid trickling back up your oesophagus and it leaves a bad taste in your mouth. Vigorous exercise that involves jumping or running can also be uncomfortable. Sports drinks and gels might aggravate your symptoms, so experiment if you want to use these.

WHAT CAN YOU DO ABOUT IT?

Eating regular, healthy meals will help. You might find that more frequent smaller meals are better than the traditional three large ones. Smoking, alcohol, spicy foods and coffee are known triggers but it's worth keeping an eye out for other foods that exacerbate your symptoms; many of my patients can't eat tomatoes or oranges.

Always allow enough time for food to be digested before exercising; for most of us this is about two hours. If you want to do exercises lying on the floor, just raising your head and shoulders slightly off the ground with a cushion or rolled-up towel can be helpful. Avoid head-down positions if they trigger any symptoms.

If dietary changes haven't helped, there are medications which are very effective.

Public toilet access

If you have a medical condition or disability that means you need to get to a toilet quickly you have two options in the UK. First, you can apply for a special key from Disability UK to allow access to over 9,000 toilets. Secondly, you can apply for a 'toilet card' from numerous charities which will explain to shop owners or others waiting why you need to access a toilet or go straight to the front of the queue. Website details can be found at the back of the book.

Some coat and protect the lining of the stomach and oesophagus from the acids, others neutralise the acid or actually stop the acid-producing cells from making the acid in the first place. Many of these can be bought over the counter, so have a chat with the pharmacist to see which would be best for you.

See your GP if: you're taking treatment for reflux but it isn't helping your symptoms ▪ you're using over-the-counter reflux medications more than once a week ▪ you're vomiting with your symptoms, have abdominal pain or you're losing weight.

Nausea and vomiting during racing and training

Pre-race nerves make everyone feel queasy, you might even retch or vomit. Trying to remain calm by working through some practised pre-race rituals can help this. Feeling sick during an endurance event is common; you might also get heartburn or upper abdominal pain.

If you're using sports supplements such as gels, make sure you dilute them with the stated amount of water because the sudden large sugar load can make you feel sick or vomit.

Nausea and vomiting lead to dehydration and being dehydrated can make you feel sick too, so it's vital to make sure you've practised your race-day drinking. Don't forget to adapt to the weather conditions as the risk of dehydration is higher on a hot day.

Avoid taking non-steroidal anti-inflammatory medications such as aspirin and ibuprofen if you struggle with nausea and vomiting. They can irritate the lining of the oesophagus and stomach; paracetamol is a safer choice if you need to take a painkiller (turn to Chapter 14 to read about pain relief for exercise).

I'm sure you've heard the opinion that 'you haven't trained hard enough unless you've vomited'. Excessive effort makes your adrenalin levels surge, halting digestion, and you often feel the effect of this after you've crossed the finish line and suddenly stopped. A lap of honour will slowly decrease your effort and help avoid this. Thankfully you don't need to train to the point of vomiting to train effectively, and repeatedly pushing yourself until you're sick isn't to be recommended.

The 'tips for troubled tummies' earlier in this chapter are just as valid for vomiting as they are for diarrhoea and you can consider using the medications mentioned in the acid reflux section too.

Piles (haemorrhoids)

About half of us will experience piles at some point in our lives; probably following

What is a stitch?

The honest answer is we don't really know what causes that horrible pain you often get in your side, usually the right side, during exercise. There are many theories, including a lack of blood supply to the diaphragm, swelling of the liver and under-breathing. Stitches tend to happen less often as you get fitter. Making sure you've left enough time for food to be digested and warming up well can prevent them. If you get one, try slowing down and breathing more deeply. Many runners say that if their stitch is on their right side, if they slow their pace and exhale as their left foot hits the ground the stitch eases. Stopping and touching your toes or running with your hands on your head are other tricks to try. Stitches are painful but harmless and will eventually go.

childbirth or when we're elderly. They don't always cause problems but sometimes they itch, bleed and make passing a bowel motion an agonising experience.

WHAT ARE THEY?

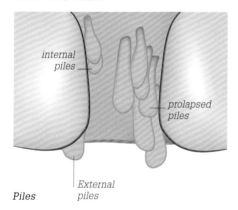

internal piles

prolapsed piles

External piles

Piles

Piles are small swellings that develop either around or just inside the anus. The swelling consists of blood vessels and fleshy tissue which form into a lump. This tends to happen when the pressure in the blood vessels has increased, so piles are more likely after giving birth or if you get constipated and sit straining on the toilet. There seems to be a genetic link making some people more susceptible than others.

The pile can originate from the tissue high up in the anal canal and stay tucked away inside; this is called an internal pile. The pile can extend and poke out (prolapse) through the anus or originate from the tissue just outside the anus, and we call these external piles.

HOW DO THEY INTERFERE WITH EXERCISE?

Having swollen lumps at your anus can be very uncomfortable and annoying when you're trying to exercise. Even walking can be sore and sitting on a bike saddle may be out of the question. Gravity can make the swellings worse, so if you've been on your feet all day, piles start to throb and get more painful. Training for an endurance event like a marathon can trigger piles, simply due to the hours spent on your feet and the extra pressure this causes on your back passage. Lifting weights can also increase this pressure. Piles can be very itchy and if you're sweaty during and after a workout this can aggravate them. Some piles never bleed but others bleed frequently; chafing during exercise might cause this. It might be the odd spot of blood in your pants or when you wipe your bottom, or an alarming gush.

WHAT CAN YOU DO ABOUT THEM?

Piles will usually go away on their own or at least shrivel and shrink until they don't cause any problems. There are a range of products to help soothe and settle these painful lumps and ease any itching. A pharmacist can advise you on which would be best for you to use. Avoiding constipation is vital. Dehydration can result in constipation so if you're training you need to make sure you drink plenty of fluids before, during and after exercise. Don't forget that exercise is a great cure for constipation as it stimulates the bowel, so if you're a pile sufferer then regular exercise is beneficial. If you're lifting heavy weights, make sure you've had proper instruction on breathing and lifting techniques because holding your breath and straining against a weight will increase pressure in the blood vessels around the anus.

Faecal incontinence

All of us have probably leaked faeces when we've had a diarrhoea bug or forcefully broken wind, but 1 per cent of people leak stools every day, and are usually suffering in silence. This tricky problem often happens alongside constipation, diarrhoea, IBS, IBD or even severe piles. Treating the underlying condition can help to resolve it. It's also a problem if you have a weak pelvic floor. Sometimes the leakage is due to poorly functioning nerves which control the anal sphincter or weakness of the sphincter itself. It can be hard to find the courage to discuss this problem with a GP, but treatments are available and the impact of a leaky bowel on everyday life, let alone on exercise, is immeasurable.

Check that your choice of underwear and clothes isn't going to make your piles worse. Keep the area as clean and dry as possible to reduce the risk of infections. Shower soon after exercise, gently pat the piles dry and apply a pile cream. Babies' nappy creams can be very useful both before and after exercise as they act as a barrier to protect the delicate skin.

See your GP if: you notice a swelling at your anus that hasn't gone after a couple of weeks or has become painful • you have any bleeding from your bottom, even if you think you have piles • you struggle with frequent constipation • you have piles and they aren't responding to treatment. There are surgical options for the most severe cases.

Bowel cancer

When we talk about bowel cancer we're mainly talking about cancer of the large bowel (colon) or rectum. Also known as colorectal cancer, it's the third most common cancer in women in the UK with approximately 18,000 women being given the diagnosis each year.

Many things increase your risk of bowel cancer, including getting older. Your risk is higher if you have immediate family members who've had bowel cancer, especially if they were under age 45 at diagnosis. There are a few inherited conditions and other cancers that can increase your risk, and if you've had inflammatory bowel disease or diabetes for many years these too may make bowel cancer more likely.

You can't change most of these risk factors but the good news is that there do seem to be many lifestyle factors that can influence your risk and you can certainly change these. The European Prospective Investigation Into Cancer (EPIC) study has been following half a million people from all over Europe for 15 years to give vital information about what factors might influence a person's risk of cancer. It's thought that up to 50 per cent of colorectal cancers could be prevented by lifestyle changes such as diet and exercise. That's a startling figure and one that should spur everyone into action, particularly if you have an increased risk from other factors.

DIET AND BOWEL CANCER

A diet which is high in fibre seems to have the lowest risk of bowel cancer. Including fibre in your daily diet in the form of wholegrain cereals or pulses is a good way to achieve this. Plenty of fruit and vegetables are important too, as they're fibrous and packed full of anti-oxidants, which have a role to play in cancer reduction, especially green, leafy, folate containing vegetables like spinach, kale and broccoli. There's good

I got piles after my second baby was born; it was a long labour. They just wouldn't go away. I was determined to pretend they didn't exist so just pushed on with a long bike ride. How I wish I'd thought about my knickers! I didn't want a VPL with my lycra so I'd put on a thong. The combination of sweat, piles, a hard saddle and tight elastic was an agonising mistake I won't make again. Nina, mum of two, road cyclist and lover of sensible pants

evidence that a diet low in red and processed meats like ham, sausages and bacon will reduce risk. Replacing them with white meat such as chicken and fish is beneficial. The jury is out on whether dairy products affect your risk: milk may decrease your risk and cheese may increase it, but more studies need to be done. The link with alcohol is clear, higher alcohol intake means a higher risk of bowel cancer. This might seem like a lengthy list of instructions but really, it all boils down to a sensible, varied, healthy diet, so don't get bogged down with the details and just enjoy lots of fresh food and make healthy choices.

OBESITY, EXERCISE AND BOWEL CANCER

Being overweight or obese will increase the risk of colon cancer by 13 per cent in the UK. Rectal cancer rates are slightly higher if you're obese but the link isn't as strong as the one with cancer of the colon. Exercising regularly is a powerful way to reduce your colon cancer risk. Studies have shown that you can reduce your risk by as much as 30–50 per cent compared to inactive people if you increase the number of times you exercise, how long you exercise and how hard too. We aren't sure yet of the benefits on rectal cancer risk. The benefits of exercise are separate to any benefits from the weight loss that may occur with exercise. Exercising during any cancer treatment is beneficial and if you've had bowel cancer then exercising regularly may help prevent the cancer recurring by as much as 50 per cent.

See your GP if: you're having recurrent abdominal pains ▪ you pass any blood in your stools ▪ your bowel habit has changed and is either more or less frequent, with constipation or diarrhoea, and this has persisted for six weeks ▪ you feel you aren't emptying your bowel properly after you've finished on the toilet ▪ you're losing weight without good reason.

Case history

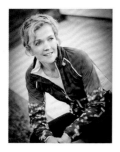

SARAH RUSSELL, REHABILITATION, BIOMECHANICS AND RUNNING COACH, WRITER, INTERNATIONAL ROWER AND TRIATHLETE, MUM OF TWO

Sarah had to have emergency surgery in 2012 when her bowel perforated as a result of a condition called diverticulitis. She needed five operations and she now has an ileostomy. This is where the bowel is diverted to the skin of the abdomen, through an opening called a stoma, through which faeces pass and are collected in a bag, rather than making their way along the rest of the digestive tract. I asked Sarah how having a stoma has impacted on her love of exercise.

'I've tried to see my stoma as a challenge to overcome, rather than a barrier to prevent me doing things. It's more "how can I work around that problem?" rather than "Oh, I can't do that because of my stoma". Of course it's not always easy, but having this conscious attitude has really helped me cope.

'I've had to work hard to rehabilitate after each operation and to rebuild my body from rock bottom. It's been both a physical and emotional journey, but gradually I've gotten stronger, fitter and more confident. In 2014 (two years after my last surgery) I became the first person with an ileostomy to run the Himalayan 100 – a hundred-mile stage race over five days at altitude in the Indian Himalaya. I got to witness the stunning sight of Mt Everest at dawn, with the first glimmers of light shining on the world's highest peak. It was breathtaking – spine-tingling stuff. When I came home from that race I felt invincible – if I can do that and survive, I thought, then I can do anything. It was incredibly empowering. Richard Nixon once said, "Only if you have been in the deepest valley can you truly appreciate the magnificence of the highest mountain." I often wonder if I'd have enjoyed it so much if I'd not experienced the "deepest valley". I doubt it. Adversity teaches us so much. It makes us stronger and shouldn't be feared. I'm actually grateful for my experience and what it's taught me. For me my stoma is simply a challenge to overcome – much like a marathon or any other race. It's not a barrier, nor is it a disability and I'm not about to let it stop me doing anything.'

Chapter 10

THE SKIN

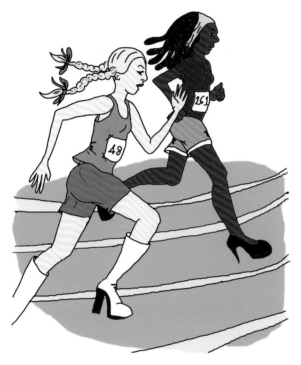

'I don't care about blisters – I just want this world record!'
A German teenager holds the world record for running 100 metres in a pair of heels; 14.531 seconds, which is just 5 seconds slower than Usain Bolt's record of 9.8 seconds

It's easy to dismiss skin problems as minor and something that won't affect our ability to exercise. The reality is that even the smallest of niggles can be a game-changer and some skin conditions are far from trivial. Skin not only holds us together but protects what's underneath. It keeps out infection, helps control body temperature and it's waterproof. It also gets rid of toxins, makes vitamin D and allows us to touch and feel. Understanding our skin, knowing how to look after it and being aware of the issues some of us face are helpful and important topics for keeping all of us active.

Skin structure

The skin is your largest organ and if you stretched it out on the floor it would cover about 1.6 square metres. Its thickness varies; for example, the skin on your eyelids is only half a millimetre thick, whereas on the soles of your feet or your back it can be ten times thicker.

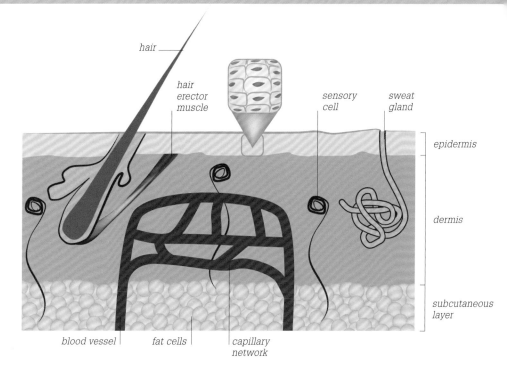

hair

hair
erector
muscle

sensory
cell

sweat
gland

epidermis

dermis

subcutaneous
layer

blood vessel   fat cells   capillary
network

The structure of skin

The skin is made up of three layers. The first is the epidermis, the thin layer on the top. At the base of this layer new skin cells are made and they gradually work their way up to the surface over the course of a couple of months where they eventually die and flake off. The cells which produce your skin pigment melanin are located in the epidermis. Under the epidermis lies the dermis; it's a much thicker layer. Here we'll find hair follicles, sweat and sebaceous glands, blood vessels and nerve endings. Finally, there's a layer of fat called subcutaneous fat, which acts as insulation, an energy store and also as padding.

Ageing and sun damage

Skin changes as we age, getting looser and more wrinkled. It's a common worry that doing lots of exercise, especially vigorous, will make skin sag, but there's no evidence to prove this. It's mostly due to the downward pull of gravity and your genetics which determine how elastic your skin is, and therefore how readily it will bounce back after being stretched. You can't alter gravity or your DNA but there are some things you can do to protect your skin from ageing.

Smoking damages the elastic properties of skin and regular smoking will age you prematurely.

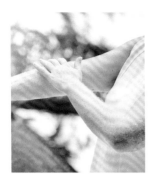

Exposure to harmful ultra violet (UV) rays from the sun can also reduce your skin's elasticity. We've all seen old ladies with thickened, leathery, wrinkled skin from years of sun damage. It's easy to take steps to protect your skin from the sun and it's important to do this all year round, especially if you regularly exercise outside. Simple measures like applying sunscreen, wearing a hat and avoiding the hottest part of the summer days are enough. Always use a sunscreen with SPF 15 or more and consider changing your usual facial moisturiser to one containing an SPF. Don't forget to protect your eyes too – invest in a good pair of sunglasses.

See your GP if: you notice any changes in a mole. This might be a change in size, shape or colour, itching, bleeding or just looking different to other moles nearby ▪ you develop any red, scaly skin lesions, particularly ones that bleed or develop a crust ▪ you have a skin sore that just doesn't seem to heal.

Common skin problems

Sometimes minor skin problems cause a whole lot of trouble when it comes to staying active. Let's look at some of the common ones and learn how to treat and prevent them.

BLISTERS

Blisters form in or just under the epidermis when skin is damaged. This is most commonly due to friction but also chemical damage, heat or extreme cold. Blisters are usually filled with clear fluid (serum) but can contain blood or pus.

Exercise as anti-ageing

Your chromosomes contain your DNA and have little protective caps at the end called telomeres. As you age, these telomeres get worn down. One of the things that shortens them is stress inside the cell. Turn back to Chapter 1 for a reminder about how being inactive causes harmful free radicals to build up in and damage cells; we call this oxidative stress. If you're physically active, there's less build-up of oxidative stress in your cells. This means less wearing down or shortening of the telomeres and therefore a slowing down of the ageing process from the inside out.

Treatment: Don't be tempted to pop blisters. The fluid is acting as a cushion to protect the delicate skin underneath and it's sterile, which means it's germ-free. Bursting them makes them susceptible to infection. They'll shrivel up on their own, when the underlying skin has healed. In the meantime, protect them with a plaster or a padded dressing. If they've burst, clean them thoroughly with warm soapy water, pat them dry and apply a sterile dressing such as a hydrocolloid blister dressing, which can be bought in any pharmacy.

Prevention: Correctly fitted shoes are vital. Go up at least half a size when buying trainers for vigorous activities to allow enough room for your toes. Check the width fitting and look for trainers with a wider toe box if necessary. All shoes take time to wear in.

Socks are just as important as shoes. You need to have the right size to prevent your toes getting squashed. Blisters develop more often in damp conditions so opt for socks made from a technical fabric which wick sweat away from the feet and dry quickly. Silk socks or liners can be a useful option if you suffer from recurrent blisters. Wool socks are great for hiking in cold weather and merino wool makes an ideal sock fabric as it's breathable and anti-bacterial for those of you with smelly feet!

Blisters aren't always on the feet, of course; gripping rackets and oars, handlebars and hand rims on wheelchairs can all cause blisters. For sports where gloves are acceptable, finding the right pair can make all the difference, and using talc or chalk can absorb moisture and prevent blistering. Altering your racket grip, changing the size or taping the handle can reduce friction. Try using a sweatband on your wrist to stop sweat running down your arm and encouraging blisters.

'Toughening up' your skin by applying surgical spirit or alcohol is controversial as it can dry skin out, leading to painful cracking and fissuring of skin instead of blisters. Applying petroleum jelly or lanolin before exercise can help and you can experiment with taping hands or feet with anti-blister tape too.

See your GP if: your blister is filled with yellow pus or has redness surrounding and spreading out from it; this suggests it's infected and might require an antibiotic.

VERRUCAS

Verrucas are warts which appear on the feet and have a flatter appearance than warts growing on your hands, because you tread on them. They're harmless but they can be uncomfortable and stop you being active.

Treatment: The majority of verrucas will go away on their own, although this may take up to two years. There's a strong argument that this allows your body to produce antibodies to the wart virus and gives you future protection against it. If a verruca is causing discomfort and you want to treat it then you can use salicylic acid to burn the verruca away. This can be bought from any pharmacy. It's a time-consuming business, as you need to soak your foot in warm water for a few minutes, file off the dead skin and apply a small amount of acid to the verruca every day for up to three months. It's effective but you need to be motivated for it to work. A quicker option is to use a freezing treatment. Freezing with liquid nitrogen used to be widely available in GP surgeries, but as the acid home treatments are cheap and effective it's rarely offered now. You can buy a home freezing spray over the counter which may not be as effective as liquid nitrogen but is another option and usually only requires one or two applications. You might want to have a try with the duct tape method; the evidence for it isn't convincing but it's easy and unlikely to cause any problems. Stick some duct tape over the verruca and once a week take it off, soak the foot in warm water and file away the dead skin with a pumice stone or soft emery board. After 12 hours reapply a new piece of tape and repeat this process for approximately eight weeks or until the verruca has gone.

Prevention: Verrucas are contagious so you can catch them by direct contact. Wearing flip flops in damp environments like communal showers or beside swimming pools can reduce your chances of catching one. If you have a verruca then you can keep swimming; covering the verruca with a waterproof plaster is adequate – there's no need for a special verruca sock. Good foot hygiene, changing socks daily and not sharing towels are other sensible steps to avoid verrucas.

See your GP if: you have multiple spreading verrucas.

CHAFING

If your exercise involves repetitive movements you might find you get sore where skin rubs against more skin or clothes. Chafed skin looks red and sometimes weeps or bleeds. The commonest areas involved are upper thighs and underarms and anywhere clothing meets the skin, such as bras straps and waistbands. Sweating can make chafing worse. Men suffer with nipple-chafing, but thankfully bras usually protect us against this.

Treatment: Chafed skin can really sting when it gets wet; it's important to make sure it's clean and dry. After drying, apply a cream containing zinc oxide (commonly used in baby's nappy creams) to soothe and protect the skin; some people prefer petroleum jelly. You might need to apply a dressing to stop more friction and discomfort, especially if you don't want a break from exercise.

Prevention: Well-fitted clothes made from technical fabrics can reduce chafing. Lycra shorts stop thighs rubbing together and clothes with smooth seams are a good choice. It helps to apply large amounts of a skin lubricant like petroleum jelly before exercise to areas that are likely to rub. This is particularly wise if you're doing an endurance event or an activity when you're going to get wet, as wet skin chafes more easily.

See your GP if: your chafed skin won't heal despite the above measures, or it's getting sticky or smells strongly.

SWEATING

How much you sweat is determined by the number of sweat glands in your dermis and how much they produce. Sweat is mainly water with some salts such as sodium, potassium and chloride; that's why it tastes salty and leaves a salt mark on your clothes after it's dried. The sweat glands in certain areas of the body, like under the arms, produce a slightly thicker type of sweat. Sweat doesn't smell; it's when it meets the bacteria on skin that the odour starts. It's easy to assume that if you increase your fitness you'll sweat less but very often the opposite is true. Sweating is one of the mechanisms your body uses to cool you down and for some, getting fitter means your body gets more efficient at losing heat and you actually sweat more.

There's a condition called hyperhidrosis where people sweat excessively. There's often an underlying medical condition, but for one type of hyperhidrosis (primary focal hyperhidrosis) there's no obvious reason; it may be genetic. It usually affects the underarms, palms, soles of the feet or head and can have a huge impact on people's lives. Many can't contemplate exercising as they worry it'll just make them sweat more.

Treatment: Use an antiperspirant which blocks sweat pores rather than a deodorant which just masks the odour of sweat. Visit the pharmacist to ask about products containing aluminium which are 'heavy-duty' antiperspirants. Initially they should be used daily but as your condition improves you can reduce this. It's important to follow the instructions and use them correctly. If they're causing irritation of the skin, missing out a day or two and applying 1 per cent hydrocortisone cream thinly for three days will help. There are a variety of other treatments available including medications, injections

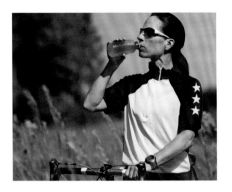

of botulinum toxin and finally surgery to remove sweat glands or divide the nerves which supply them. Don't forget that after exercise you need to replace the fluids you've lost through sweat. Sweat contains salts, so if you've been exercising heavily for over an hour then using a sports drink that contains electrolytes is an ideal way to do this.

Prevention: Although sweating is activated by the sympathetic nervous system which you can't control, you might find there are some triggers to your sweating that you can avoid, such as spicy food, caffeine and alcohol. Looser clothes are often better than tight and try experimenting with different fabrics to see what suits you best. Natural fibres are recommended, but for exercise you might find that some of the new technical fabrics which wick sweat away from the body are better.

See your GP if: the amount you sweat is affecting and restricting your daily life.

Common skin infections

We all have a range of micro-organisms living on and in our body; these include many types of bacteria and fungi. We call these 'commensals'. They're supposed to be there and they don't cause any harm; in fact, they can be beneficial, helping with many bodily functions such as digestion and immunity. However, if conditions change there can be an overgrowth of commensal bacteria or other non-commensals can invade and you develop an infection.

ATHLETE'S FOOT

This is a fungal infection and, as the name suggests, it's common if you live in your trainers. Fungi love warm, dark, moist places and where better than a well-loved sports shoe! It usually starts between the toes where skin becomes flaky and itchy. It can look red and dry or white and soggy. It can then spread across the top and bottom of the foot and make your feet smell.

Treatment: This infection usually settles quickly with good foot hygiene and a trip to the pharmacy to buy some antifungal cream, spray or powder. If your feet are really itchy, look for a preparation that contains a mild steroid like 1 per cent hydrocortisone.

Keep going with the treatment for a few days even after the condition seems to have cleared up. In resistant or very severe cases you might need to see your GP to discuss using an antifungal tablet.

Prevention: Washing and drying your feet carefully every day (including between your toes) is important but not easy when you're pushed for time and rushing to get dressed in a changing room whilst minding a baby and toddler! Change your socks daily and always after exercise. Alternating two pairs of sports shoes will ensure they dry out thoroughly between wears. Leather shoes breathe better than synthetic fabrics and you might want to invest in flip flops for communal showers and changing rooms.

INTERTRIGO

As well as dark soggy trainers, fungi and bacteria love to grow in warm skin folds. Some of us have deeper folds than others, but under breasts, in armpits, in our groins and between our buttocks are top spots. This is a particular problem if you use a wheelchair. Adding damp sweat to the mix makes an even more favourable environment for the multiplication of germs. The most common germ to grow is candida, which is a yeast or fungus. The rash is usually red, sore and can sometimes itch.

Treatment: Keep the area as clean and dry as possible. Make sure you shower soon after exercise and avoid perfumed products. You can buy antifungal creams over the counter, the same ones used for athlete's foot. These should be applied thinly twice a day after washing. The rash should start to clear up within a week and you should keep going for a few days after it seems to have gone. If you want to exercise while you have intertrigo, you can use a baby's nappy cream like Sudocrem to protect the area.

Prevention: Keeping skin clean and dry is the main defence against intertrigo. Experiment to find clothes that minimise sweating and always wash and change straight after exercise. If you're using a hair dryer, a good tip is to direct the air to any problem areas like under your breasts or between your buttocks to ensure they're absolutely dry. Avoid skin moisturisers, which can make skin soggy, but a barrier nappy cream can help if put on before exercise.

See your GP if: your rash is very weepy or crusted ▪ your rash is not clearing with antifungal creams. Sometimes bacterial infections are the cause and an antibiotic may be required.

VULVAL AND VAGINAL INFECTIONS

It can be tricky to keep a healthy balance of bacteria in the vulva and vagina. Most of us tend to over-wash, and being too clean strips away healthy bacteria. If you're very active and shower multiple times a day, you're at risk from these types of infection. The commonest infections are thrush, which is an overgrowth of candida (a type of fungus), and bacterial vaginosis (BV), where there's overgrowth of a mixture of bacteria. Both can give you a vaginal discharge; the discharge with thrush is usually white or cream in colour and sometimes lumpy like cottage cheese. BV discharge tends to be more grey in colour, and is often very smelly. Both conditions can make sex uncomfortable and both can be itchy, but thrush is usually itchier than BV.

Treatment: Candida and the bacteria causing BV are all commensals living normally on skin and if your symptoms are very mild then you might not need any treatment at all. Thrush is treated by using a pessary (tablet which is inserted into the vagina) or a tablet that you swallow. Antifungal creams can also be applied to external thrush. These can all be bought from a pharmacy. BV usually requires a trip to the GP for treatment, as you need to be prescribed an antibiotic tablet or vaginal cream.

Prevention: Both these conditions can be recurrent, often at certain times in the menstrual cycle, when you're unwell, on antibiotics or after sex; it can be hard to prevent them coming back. Washing once a day is enough, avoiding perfumed soaps, bubble baths and shower gels. Don't douche your vagina (this means vigorous washing that pushes water inside you). Biological washing powders and fabric conditioners can be a trigger so try using an extra rinse cycle on the washing machine. There are vaginal gels available over the counter and on prescription that work by correcting the pH (acid/alkali balance) in the vagina. Studies haven't shown a clear benefit to these yet, although anecdotally some women feel they help prevent recurrence. It might help to use a plain moisturiser around the vulva and vaginal area to help condition the skin.

See your GP if: you're pregnant and you have a vaginal discharge ▪ you aren't sure what's causing your vaginal discharge ▪ you've self-treated but your condition hasn't cleared ▪ you keep getting recurrent symptoms ▪ you have any bleeding associated with your discharge.

FOLLICULITIS

Skin problems in areas where hair grows are common. Hair grows out of a shaft or follicle, which gives germs a place to nestle and the environment is ideal. Folliculitis simply means inflammation (itis) of a follicle; the usual suspect is staphylococcus aureus, a bacterial skin commensal. The skin looks bumpy and red and you might see collections of yellow pus around each hair shaft called pustules. Being warm, damp and sweaty with exercise can be a trigger for folliculitis, especially in the groins and armpits. Traumatising the hair shafts and skin by shaving, plucking or waxing also makes you more susceptible to infection.

Treatment: Mild infections will often clear with simple hygiene and adding a little salt water or antiseptic to your bath. It's sensible to try an antiseptic cream or spray too. If these steps aren't helping, see your GP as you may need an antibiotic cream or tablet.

Prevention: Ideally you should wash daily and always after exercise, with a mild soap. Poorly maintained hot tubs are associated with a type of folliculitis so have a good wash with soap after a long soak in a hot tub. Change your razor blade frequently and never share blades. Try using a hair removal cream or waxing instead of shaving and it may help if you gently exfoliate beforehand.

See your GP if: you aren't sure whether your rash is folliculitis or not ▪ home treatments aren't helping ▪ your folliculitis keeps coming back.

ABSCESSES

If a follicle or skin pore gets infected it can start to swell and enlarge and a boil or abscess can quickly develop. Abscesses are usually bacterial infections and are filled with thick pus. They can look red, feel warm and be incredibly painful. Bartholin's abscesses form just at the entrance to the vagina when the Bartholin's gland, which secretes vaginal mucous, gets infected. Perianal abscesses are also common and these form in the skin close to the anus and usually originate from small anal glands.

Treatment: Small abscesses on the skin don't always need treatment and many will settle when they eventually burst. Warm baths can soften the skin and if an abscess bursts just gently wipe any pus away with clean tissue or gauze and give it a thorough wash with warm soapy water. Larger abscesses, particularly Bartholin's or perianal abscesses, may require surgical treatment. Some will settle with a course of antibiotics, but once well-established they often need to be drained. This is done using local anaesthetic to numb the skin and making an incision in the abscess to allow the contents to leak out. Larger and deeper abscesses may require a general anaesthetic. You'll need to wait until the area has fully healed up before starting to exercise again.

Prevention: Good skin care is the most important way to prevent abscesses, but for some women, even with scrupulous personal hygiene, abscesses still develop and it can often just be a case of bad luck!

See your GP if: you have a growing abscess which is becoming painful ▪ you have an abscess and feel unwell or have a high temperature ▪ you suffer with recurrent abscesses.

Nail problems

BLACK NAILS

The delicate skin underneath a nail is called the nail bed. When a nail is damaged the blood vessels on the nail bed can bleed; there's nowhere for the blood to escape to so it collects under the nail. Initially it looks red, then purple, and finally black, and the nail usually falls off. This is called a subungual haematoma, which literally means a bleed under a nail. If the damage happens suddenly, for example if a fingernail is crushed by a cricket ball, then it can be intensely painful, but if it's due to more gradual, repeated trauma such as a toenail being damaged by running then there may be no pain at all. Crush injuries involving torn nails and possible fractured fingers are best dealt with in an accident and emergency department.

Treatment: Sudden, throbbing subungual haematomas can be drained by trephining (making a small hole in the nail) to allow blood to escape. This is best done by a health professional to avoid infection developing. Black nails that aren't painful can simply be left alone. It's best to leave the nail in place for as long as possible to protect the delicate nail bed underneath. When it does fall off, a new nail will grow slowly from the bottom of the nail bed.

Prevention: Accidents happen but you can minimise the injury to toenails by allowing adequate room for your toes in your shoes and socks. See the section on blisters for advice on this. Nails are often damaged when running downhill when your foot is pushed forwards into your shoe. Experiment with different laces and lacing patterns for your trainers to minimise how much your foot slides about inside your shoe.

See your GP if: you've a single black nail that hasn't been injured and isn't resolving. Very occasionally, a black nail can be a malignant melanoma (skin cancer).

FUNGAL NAIL INFECTIONS

The same fungi that cause athlete's foot can penetrate into your nails. The nail becomes thickened, discoloured (usually yellow) and either brittle or flaky. These infections are more of a pest than a danger; the infection can spread to other nails but is harmless.

Treatment: Infected nails don't necessarily need to be treated. Frustratingly, all treatments take six to nine months to work as you have to wait for a new nail to grow. Nails can become thickened and discoloured through simple damage rather than infection so your GP may take a nail sample for testing before starting treatment. The two options for treatment are antifungal nail lacquers and oral medications. Lacquers need to be applied frequently and after filing the nail; persistence is required! Oral medications are considered if multiple nails are affected, but you need to discuss the possibility of side effects with your GP. Be aware that treatments don't always work and there's no guarantee the nail will return to a normal shape.

Prevention: Treat any athlete's foot early to stop infections spreading to nails. Damaged nails are more likely to be affected so allow enough room for your toes in your sports shoes. Avoid sharing towels and footwear and consider flip flops for changing rooms and communal showers.

See your GP if: you have multiple infected nails or your infection is causing pain or embarrassment.

Lacing up trainers

You might be sure you've got the right size shoe but still have problems with blisters, damaged nails and even foot numbness. Here are some different ways to lace up:

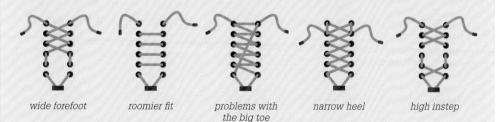

wide forefoot   roomier fit   problems with   narrow heel   high instep
                                            the big toe

Allergic to exercise

If a rash appears every time you exercise, it may be a condition called exercise-induced urticaria. Red blotches, blisters or bumps appear on your skin; they can be big or small and are often itchy. They usually go within ten minutes of stopping your activity. Speak to your GP about using antihistamine medications to prevent this happening. In extremely rare cases this can progress to a full allergic reaction and include swelling of the face and difficulty breathing, in which case you need to call an emergency ambulance.

PARONYCHIA

Paronychia is the medical term for those annoying infections you get in the skin just at the edge of your fingernails or toenails. They often happen in association with a nail which ingrows or if you nibble the skin in this area. They can be very sore and the infection can potentially become severe if it spreads to surrounding skin.

Treatment: At the first sign of a paronychia it's a good idea to start soaking the affected finger or toe at least twice a day in some warm, salty water. If the infection is mild, try using some antifungal cream from the pharmacy, as these infections are often caused by fungi. If this doesn't help or the infection is more severe and pus is building up in the skin, see your GP. You'll require antibiotics and sometimes the pus needs to be drained by lancing (making a small cut). If the condition is due to an ingrowing nail, then you may need to have this removed.

Prevention: Good hand and foot hygiene obviously helps avoid these types of skin infection. Avoid trimming your nails too short and make sure you cut them straight across rather than with a rounded edge to help prevent nails ingrowing. Damaged nails are more likely to get infected so, again, make sure your footwear fits properly.

See your GP if: you have an infection beside your nail which isn't clearing with salt-water soaks ▪ redness is spreading to the skin further down your finger or toe ▪ you're in a lot of pain with your infection.

Exercising with long-term skin conditions

Lots of us struggle with long-term conditions of our skin such as acne, rosacea, eczema and psoriasis. Exercise is a good stress reliever which can help you cope with any long-term health problem, and many women feel that regular exercise helps to keep their skin healthy, although the evidence for this is sparse. You might actually find that exercise makes your skin condition worse and that can put you off being active. It can be a real balancing act. You need to try to stop your skin being a barrier to activity so here are my top tips for exercising with skin problems.

Before exercise

◎ Consider taking off make-up before exercising. Many brands are 'non-comedogenic', which means they don't block pores, but if you wear make-up and are struggling with your skin, try removing it before you work out.

◎ Apply a light moisturiser before you exercise, particularly if you're exercising outdoors. Choose a thicker one if you're going to swim. Pay particular attention to chapped or inflamed skin that might be aggravated by cold or windy weather. It'll act as a protective barrier and stop stinging caused by salty sweat too.

◎ Apply a sunscreen with a minimum of SPF 15 and look for a very mild, unscented brand that won't irritate skin or cause stinging if sweat takes it into your eyes.

During exercise

◎ Wipe away sweat on a clean towel or sweat band and not with your hand or T-shirt.

◎ Keep your hair off your face by tying it back or wearing a headband.

◎ Wear a hat with a good brim if you suffer from rosacea and sunlight is a trigger.

◎ Experiment with different fabrics for your exercise kit; natural fibres such as cotton and loose-fitting clothes might suit you best, although technical fabrics that wick sweat away are also good.

◎ Try not to overheat; pause when you need to cool down.

◎ Drink plenty of fluids to keep yourself cool and hydrated.

After exercise

◎ Shower soon after exercise using a mild, unperfumed soap substitute. This is particularly important if you've been swimming in chlorinated water. Use a mild, anti-bacterial facewash for acne.

◎ Apply liberal amounts of your moisturiser after you've showered. Keeping skin soft and conditioned and preventing it from drying out is key for most skin conditions.

◎ Wash exercise clothes in a mild detergent. Fabric softener may irritate you, but so might harsher fabrics that haven't been conditioned. Some washing machines have a programme for sensitive skin which includes an extra rinse cycle.

My acne has never affected my confidence to exercise, although there was one time it came pretty close! It was really horrendous: my face was literally covered in spots and I didn't want to go to my dance class as I was embarrassed, but I decided to go after all. The people in my dance class are among the very few who'll say to me: 'Your skin's looking a lot better now.' I'd actually like people to acknowledge my bad skin, but nobody ever does. I think they don't want to upset me, but it makes me feel like I'm invisible when they don't mention it.   Sarah, mum of three, runner who loves to dance

I've had rosacea for 14 years, since I was 28. Exercise, stress, sunlight, spicy food, heat, cold and alcohol make it flare up. It's the redness that really gets to me; antibiotics clear the spots but nothing works on the redness of my cheeks, so I use a moisturiser which has a green tint to it which takes the edge off the redness, and a lightweight camouflage cream when I don't want to wear make-up.   Kara, mum of six from Poole

Cellulite

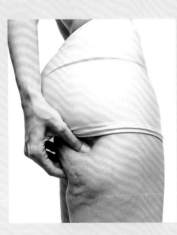

Cellulite is simply fatty tissue under the skin, usually around the hips, thighs and bottom. You don't have to be overweight to have cellulite; it can affect even the skinniest of women. It's largely an issue of genetics, so if you've got cellulite your female relatives probably have too. The deposits of fat put tension on the connective tissue (the skeleton of skin) and that causes the classic lumpy, dimpled look. It can be hard to shift. It seems much less responsive to the usual fat-busting diets and exercises than other areas of fat deposition.

Nothing you can rub on will magically dissolve the fat. Expensive massage and surgical techniques may provide only a temporary improvement in appearance. Some women do shed cellulite, though, and report that a mixture of cardio and strength-training exercise and a healthy diet are the best routes to success.

Chapter 11

FEELING TIRED ALL THE TIME

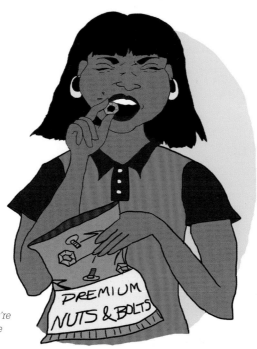

My doctor told me to eat more nuts as they're full of iron, but they're ruining my teeth

One of the most common issues women come to see me about is feeling tired all the time (TATT). It's a really tricky one to unravel as many medical problems can present with tiredness. It's not unusual to end up having a batch of blood tests to check for underlying disorders, but actually, it's rare for anything to show up. It's much more likely that lifestyle is to blame. We shouldn't really be surprised if we're always tired, considering the amount most of us try to pack into each day. The ongoing pressures of everyday life can be exhausting and it's unrealistic to think that this won't take its toll on us. Feeling TATT is another of our body's warning signs; it's trying to let us know we need to give a bit of attention to ourselves.

Finding the time and energy to exercise is often a big challenge but exercise can be a useful strategy for dealing with tiredness. It can help you cope with the day-to-day stresses that are wearing you out, it can energise you and help to ensure you have a

Specialist opinion

KATE PERCY, COOK, MUM OF THREE, SERIAL MARATHON RUNNER AND AUTHOR OF GO FASTER FOOD AND GO FASTER FOOD FOR KIDS WWW.GOFASTERFOOD.COM

Eating for energy

In the melee of daily life, work and family commitments it can be all too easy to get by on ready meals, the kids' leftovers, or even just forget to eat! Before I discovered how the right nutrition could have such an enormous effect on my energy levels, I would rush to work on scraps of the children's toast (the discarded crusts of course!) and would often miss lunch. By the evening I'd sometimes feel as if all energy had been sucked out of me. The mere thought of exercise was a struggle. That's no way to live! What, when and how we eat is not only the starting block to better energy levels, it's also the key to our whole wellbeing.

Try these simple guidelines to boost your vitality:

◎ Eat a variety of foods from each food group – carbohydrate, protein and fats – focusing on unrefined, slow-release, fresh and natural foods, including lots of wholegrains, vegetables, pulses and beans, fruit, lean meat and fish, eggs and foods containing healthy fats such as avocados and salmon.

◎ Keep well-hydrated throughout the day.

◎ Swap processed, fatty foods and those high in refined sugar for healthier options - try fresh fruit or energy-dense nuts and seeds instead of your mid-morning chocolate biscuit, sweet potatoes instead of chips, wholegrain instead of white bread.

Incorporate eating and drinking properly into your daily routine. That doesn't necessarily mean slaving over a hot stove for hours on end. A good start is to get your mornings and evenings sorted; a proper breakfast such as porridge or poached egg on wholemeal toast and a decent evening meal; a stir fry with chicken and lots of fresh vegetables, pasta with homemade pesto or a sweet potato omelette, for instance; all excellent 'quick-fixes' packed with the right nutrients to sustain energy. With a little planning you can make wholesome snack bars and batches of soup and stews in advance. It's also a great idea to keep a healthy stash of store-cupboard foods so that there's always a stand-by meal to be made. If, like me, you're not a planner, build in time for a quick visit to the shop every day, perhaps on your way home from work or the school run, so there's always something fresh to cook in the evening.

good night's sleep. You're more robust and productive if you're in good physical and mental shape and exercise can help you achieve this by giving you a feeling of wellbeing.

Lifestyle and fatigue

Sometimes you need to go back to basics of eating and sleeping to improve your energy levels. You need to make sure you're eating properly. Have a look at the eating for energy tips from Kate Percy.

Adequate sleep can be difficult or impossible to achieve with a hectic life or young children. Sometimes you need to just do the best you can to get through the day and not aim for perfection. Turn to Chapter 5 for advice on how to exercise with young children, or follow the sleep tips below if little ones aren't the cause of your sleep deprivation.

Making time for yourself must become a priority. You can't constantly give to others and not take anything back; 'me time' is underestimated as a tool to fight fatigue. Delegate and be pro-active in making sure you have some time every week which is yours and yours alone. It should be the last thing in the diary to be cancelled, not the first. It's crucial in helping you to stay strong and energised and able to cope. You may need to ask others for help to achieve this time and if it involves child care then you may need to pay to get it. Use that time however you want, but using it to exercise is a clever way to get the benefit of the time but also the health boost of activity. Turn to Chapter 17 for tips on fitting exercise into a busy day.

SOMETIMES IT'S OK NOT TO EXERCISE

It's easy for exercise itself to become stressful, especially if you're following a rigorous training programme or have a particular goal in mind. You need to assess whether you're just lacking motivation and need a push out of the door or whether you're

Since starting to exercise regularly I've found I'm more productive around my home. When I can squeeze a run or quick high-intensity workout into my day I seem to have lots of energy and can get through my daily chores more quickly and efficiently. Kirstin Poppleton, mum to two boys, Lancashire

I've just had a really long week at work. It was either go for a pint or go for a run. I chose the run and do you know what? It worked; I feel so much better. Jo Callaghan, secretary and mum of two

Top tips for a good night's sleep

If you're one of those people who find it hard to sleep or is always tired try these tips for a peaceful, restorative night.

- Establish a strict routine so you go to bed and get up at the same time each day. Use an alarm clock and, crucially, stick to the routine at weekends too.
- Don't nap in the day. If you feel like dropping off after a meal then get up, move about or go out for a walk. If you must nap then only allow 20 minutes, no later than early afternoon.
- Make sure you've had plenty of exercise and fresh air during the day so you're physically as well as mentally tired. Avoid vigorous exercise before bed if you find it too stimulating.
- Make your bedroom a relaxing haven. Don't work in there or watch TV. Tidy away mess so it's a calm environment.
- Keep your bedroom dark and don't overheat it.
- Avoid stimulants like alcohol and caffeine from 4pm onwards (yes, sadly that includes chocolate).
- Don't eat your main meal too close to bed time; allow at least three hours for digestion.
- Allow two hours of screen-free time before bed; don't look at your phone in bed, turn off social media and forget about your emails.
- Find an activity that helps you unwind before bed; a soak in the bath, reading a book or listening to music.
- Keep a notebook and pen by your bed; then, when you can't sleep, take those racing thoughts out of your head and write them down in the notebook. Random words and irrational feelings are fine. You can look at them and rationalise them in the morning.
- Learn relaxation techniques to send you off to sleep. There are lots of CDs and apps to help with this.
- If you can't sleep or you wake in the night and can't get back to sleep don't allow yourself to get frustrated; stay calm. Lying peacefully is still regenerative for your body and mind.
- If you haven't dropped off after half an hour, get up but don't reward yourself with an activity you enjoy. Do something mundane such as ironing or tidying. Don't drink a stimulant like a cup of tea. Try warm milk or water and after half an hour return to bed and try the relaxation techniques again.

overdoing it and are in need of a rest. Learning to listen to your body and pace yourself is vital. If you push too hard you can end up injured, ill or exhausted. This can be particularly true as you age or if you have health problems; it takes longer to recover and adequate rest is more important. You might not feel 100 per cent if you're coming down with an illness or if you have a flare-up of an ongoing medical problem. You need to become an expert in your own body and listen to your intuition about what's right for you. Sometimes a day or a week off exercise is what you need and that should be taken without guilt. Don't forget that exercise doesn't have to be vigorous to be beneficial and gentler activities like walking are good for you too. Learning to adapt what you do to how you feel is a crucial skill that takes time to learn but can help you stay active and healthy throughout your life.

Medical causes of fatigue

Lifestyle is usually the cause of fatigue but sometimes there are medical reasons to explain why you're feeling tired all the time. Anaemia and thyroid disorders are the most common, and extreme tiredness can be due to chronic fatigue syndrome. Let's have a look at these in more detail.

ANAEMIA

Red blood cells are made in the marrow deep in your bones. The marrow is constantly manufacturing new red blood cells as they only last about 100 days. Red cells contain haemoglobin, which attaches to oxygen; their main function is to transport this oxygen around your body from your lungs to your tissues and organs. Anaemia means there are low levels of red blood cells and in order to deliver enough oxygen to your muscles your body has to work harder, so you may have a faster pulse or breathing rate if you're

I've learnt about pacing myself the hard way! I've discovered that high-impact sports don't suit my joint problems. I don't exercise every day either: walking for 45 minutes three days a week is perfect for me. Sometimes I'll do several gentle workout sessions through the day instead of a walk, including lots of trips up and down our stairs. Some weeks I do almost nothing. My body needs a rest, and I'm learning not to feel guilty about it. Now, if I'm really tired, I'm better at recognising the necessity of stopping. I'm not ashamed to admit that there are occasions when turning over in bed and going back to sleep is absolutely the right choice. Sarah, artist with chronic pain anaemic. You might feel dizzy or lightheaded and it's common to feel really tired. If you notice a change in your ability to exercise, if you're more out of breath than usual and lacking in energy, it's worth considering whether you may be anaemic.

Causes of anaemia   You can become anaemic if you're not making enough red blood cells or if you're using them up too quickly. Problems with bone marrow are thankfully rare so low production is usually simply due to a lack of ingredients. The commonest cause of anaemia in the UK is iron deficiency. Iron is vital for red blood cell production and diets today commonly don't contain enough of it. You might eat it, but conditions like coeliac disease or inflammatory bowel disease can stop it being absorbed properly from your gut. With iron deficiency anaemia you might find you're itchy or your hair's falling out. Have a look at the 'eating for iron' tips later in this chapter to find out how to increase your iron intake. These are particularly useful if you're pregnant, as your iron requirements go up and it's common to become iron deficient in pregnancy. Vitamin B12 and folate are also needed for red cell production; deficiencies in these are less common and usually due to absorption problems and hereditary conditions.

Anaemia can also happen if you're losing red blood cells more quickly than you're making them. This might be an obvious loss like heavy periods but the blood loss might be subtle and unnoticed such as hidden blood in your stools caused by a bowel cancer. This is why it's a good idea to see a GP if you think you're anaemic, rather than just taking an iron supplement.

Foot-strike haemolysis

Red blood cells can be destroyed if they're damaged and there's an interesting condition called foot-strike haemolysis. The theory is that by marching or running long distances red blood cells are compressed and destroyed when your foot hits the ground. A study from 2003 compared runners to cyclists and whilst both groups experienced some red cell damage, foot strike was concluded to be the major contributor to the damage in the runners. Another study in 2012 looked at runners who had completed a 60-kilometre ultra-marathon and conversely found that damage from foot-strike was unlikely to be significant. It remains an area of controversy, and it's also not clear what role shoe type or terrain has to play in this condition. If you're covering large numbers of miles on foot it makes sense to be alert to the potential risk of anaemia.

Treating anaemia First you need to see your GP to establish the underlying cause for your anaemia. Perhaps you need to look at ways to reduce your heavy periods or you may need some further investigations. If you're lacking in vitamin B12 or folate, your GP will advise you on supplementation. If iron deficiency is the cause of your anaemia you must take steps to increase your iron intake through your diet and you might also need to take an iron supplement. Some people find iron tablets make them constipated, nauseated or that they cause abdominal pain or diarrhoea. If this is the case, try taking them with food. These symptoms usually settle down, but if they don't, speak to your GP about reducing the dose or trying a different formula. Iron supplements need to be taken for several months to reverse the anaemia and then build up the body's iron stores again.

Exercising with anaemia You can become anaemic so gradually that your body gets used to it and you don't notice any effect on your exercise tolerance. Conversely, if your red blood cell level drops quickly you can be acutely aware of the symptoms and exercising can be very unpleasant and difficult. There's no strict level at which exercising is safe or unsafe. It's more a case of how much strain it's putting on your body and how it makes you feel. If you're out of breath with a racing pulse and feeling lightheaded when you exercise, then of course you should stop. You might need to cut back to gentle activities while being treated for anaemia. It can take several weeks for blood levels to return to normal but then you'll usually feel a lot better and less fatigued by exercise.

HYPOTHYROIDISM – UNDERACTIVE THYROID

The thyroid gland sits in the neck and plays a vital role in controlling your metabolism. Hypothyroidism is a common medical problem affecting two in 100 people in the UK

Giving blood and exercising

Don't do vigorous exercise just before giving blood and avoid it for the rest of the day after you've donated too. The following day it's fine to exercise if you feel OK, but bear in mind it can take six to 12 weeks for your haemoglobin levels to return to normal so you might not perform at your best. For this reason, don't donate just prior to an important sporting event; instead, give blood afterwards during recovery.

Specialist opinion

KATE PERCY, COOK, MUM OF THREE, SERIAL MARATHON RUNNER AND AUTHOR OF GO FASTER
FOOD AND GO FASTER FOOD FOR KIDS WWW.GOFASTERFOOD.COM

EATING FOR IRON

Women who are menstruating need a significantly higher amount of iron in their diets
(14.8mg/day) than their male counterparts (8.7mg/day) predominantly because they need to
replenish iron lost through bleeding.

Haem iron is found in meat and eating two portions a week such as lean steak, venison,
liver, the dark meat on duck, turkey or chicken, eggs, shellfish such as oysters, mussels and
clams and to a lesser extent oily fish will boost your iron levels. Pregnant women, however,
should avoid liver due to its high levels of vitamin A. Spaghetti with mussels or clams,
parsley and garlic is a low-fat meal packed with iron and sustaining carbohydrate. Or try
venison steak, which is low in fat; griddle it like a fillet steak and serve with steamed kale
drizzled with walnut oil.

Non-haem iron is found in vegetarian foods such as beans and pulses, green leafy
vegetables, dried fruit (especially apricots), nuts and wholegrain cereals or iron-fortified
bread and breakfast cereals. These contain fibre and substances called phytates and tannins
that bind the iron into compounds, making it harder for the body to get at. However,
combining non-haem sources with foods that are rich in vitamin C (such as green leafy
vegetables, tomatoes or fruit juice) can enhance the absorption. Tea and coffee will inhibit
absorption so avoid drinking these at the same time as a meal. Vegetarian iron-boosting
meals include lentil dhal with fresh ginger and heaps of coriander, a spinach or kale salad
with toasted walnuts, chickpea falafel or, plain and simple, a mushroom omelette.

Don't forget, too, that some of the best treats come packed with iron! Try dark chocolate,
chocolate-coated nuts and raisins, chocolate tiffin, and sweet medjhool dates.

and it's 10 times more common in women than men. You're more likely to be affected as
you get older and it often begins around the time of the menopause or after childbirth.
On a global scale, the commonest cause of hypothyroidism is iodine deficiency. In
developed countries, however, this is rare, as we have plenty of iodine in our diets,
much of it in the form of iodised salt; hypothyroidism is usually due to an autoimmune
condition, and it's often hereditary.

I've suffered from severe anaemia for as long as I can remember, largely thanks to a very rare condition called hereditary hemorrhagic telangiectasia (HHT) which causes several nose bleeds a week – not ideal for an endurance runner! At its worst my haemoglobin (Hb) was 5.7 (it should be between 12 and 15). I remember the fire alarm went off at work and I had to climb the stairs back to my desk. I actually thought I wasn't going to make it as I clutched the balcony, gasping for breath, my head spinning with stars. That was a few years ago and things are a little better now, but I am and always will be permanently anaemic despite iron tablets and intravenous iron infusions. It's not ideal and accepting that my training and performance will always be curtailed is not easy but there are worse cards to be dealt. I always know when my Hb is dipping below 9, as high-intensity work becomes almost impossible. Everything feels just horrendously hard, way harder than a normal hill or speed session. The only thing I can liken it to is hitting the marathon wall; your body just has nothing more to give. Constant fatigue is a problem and every cell in my body can hurt as it tries to get oxygen from somewhere. When my Hb is in a more normal range, running feels like a gift and a real joy, and I feel I could carry on forever. This rarely happens so I make the most of those highs! Shona Thomson, adventure marathon runner

Symptoms The symptoms of an underactive thyroid can be hard to spot as they're numerous, common and often start and progress very slowly. You might feel tired and unrefreshed by sleep. You might gain weight, despite having a poor appetite, and suffer with constipation. Sometimes skin and hair become very dry and hair may start to thin or fall out. It's really common to feel cold all the time and to generally feel 'slowed up' in your thinking and functioning. You might notice a swelling at the front of your neck called a goitre; this isn't present in all types of hypothyroidism. If hypothyroidism progresses and is left untreated for many years, it can become serious.

Diagnosis and treatment It's routine for a GP to check your thyroid function if you are suffering with significant tiredness and blood tests are usually all that's needed to make the diagnosis of hypothyroidism. The hormones that are trying to stimulate the thyroid gland are high and the thyroid hormones themselves are low because the gland isn't functioning properly. Sometimes, however, it's not as clear cut as this and you may have a gland that is being heavily stimulated but is still managing to produce a normal

Iron stores

Your body keeps a store of iron to use when your blood iron levels drop. It stores it as ferritin inside cells in your liver, and a smaller amount in your muscles, spleen and bone marrow. A blood test to check ferritin levels gives a good indication of how much iron you have stored away. You'll usually have a low ferritin level if you have iron-deficiency anaemia but you may not have got to that stage and a low ferritin level may simply indicate that you're on the way to becoming anaemic and need to take action to increase your iron intake. Interestingly, a study published in the BMJ in 2003 found that women complaining of fatigue who were not anaemic, but had low ferritin levels, felt their tiredness improved after four weeks of taking an iron supplement. A further study in France in 2006 confirmed this. Whilst iron is not always pleasant to take, if you're feeling very tired and your ferritin levels are low there's evidence to prove that a course of iron may well improve your symptoms.

level of hormones. This is called 'subclinical hypothyroidism' and it often progresses to full hypothyroidism. A repeat blood test every three to six months and a discussion with your GP will determine whether you need treatment.

Treatment involves taking a daily dose of thyroid hormone as a tablet. Follow-up blood tests are required to make sure you're taking the right dose. It can be harmful to take excess thyroid replacement therefore blood testing is imperative.

HYPERTHYROIDISM – OVERACTIVE THYROID

Hyperthyroidism is a less common diagnosis than hypothyroidism, but it still affects one in 100 people in the UK and is six times more common in women than in men. It usually needs specialist assessment and treatment. An overactive thyroid gland tends to make you feel 'speeded up', twitchy, shaky and irritable. Despite this 'speeding up', you can feel excessively tired. It can be hard to concentrate or sit still and you can lose weight unintentionally. Sweating, palpitations and sleep disturbance are also common You might develop a thyroid swelling in your neck called a goitre or thyroid eye disease where eyes become uncomfortable, appear to be bulging and vision can be affected. It's usually due to an autoimmune condition called Grave's disease, but can also be caused by non-cancerous tumours in the gland, called nodules. Treatments include drugs to ease the symptoms and anti-thyroid drugs to slow down thyroid hormone production. Sometimes a radioactive iodine is given to destroy the gland, and finally surgery to remove all or part of the gland may be offered.

Chronic fatigue

Chronic fatigue, also known as myalgic encephalomyelitis (ME), is a poorly understood condition where fatigue becomes extreme, lasts for over four months and interferes so much with daily life that those affected are unable to live a normal existence. We don't know what causes it, whether it's triggered by genetics, an infection, or whether the immune system is to blame. It's an area needing more research and sufferers and carers are desperate for answers. Along with the feelings of tiredness, you might experience headaches, muscle pains and bowel symptoms. It's not unusual to feel dizzy or have problems balancing, and an oversensitivity to light or noise. Sleep can be fitful and unrefreshing. Any exertion is followed by increased tiredness and a sense that you're 'paying for it' in the days afterwards.

Recovery from chronic fatigue takes time but is possible. Treatment focuses on sleep management and periods of rest. Therapies such as cognitive behavioural therapy (CBT) and graded exercise therapy (GET) can be useful but must be supervised by a specially trained therapist. GET involves very gradually increasing the time spent being physically active, at a low level. Once this can be maintained for 30 minutes the aim is to slowly increase the intensity. It may take months or even years to achieve and setbacks are common, so it's hard to stay motivated. It's a complex condition requiring very individualised approaches because, yet again, we are all different.

Other causes of fatigue

Whilst anaemia, thyroid disorders and chronic fatigue are important medical causes of fatigue, there are many others. We mustn't forget that chronic (long-term) pain is exhausting. Many medications can also have the side effect of making you feel tired. Health conditions such as diabetes, coeliac, kidney and heart disease are all associated with tiredness. It can be difficult to know how much fatigue is normal and acceptable.

See your GP if: you're losing or gaining weight with no obvious cause ▪ you're having night sweats and you aren't menopausal ▪ your periods are heavy ▪ your bowel habit has changed, you've had blood in your stools, abdominal pain or recurrent bloating ▪ you're more out of breath than normal or you're getting palpitations, dizziness or chest pains ▪ you notice any lumps or bumps in your neck, arm pits, groins or breasts ▪ you're excessively thirsty or you're passing lots more urine than normal ▪ your tiredness is excessive, interfering with daily life, and nothing helps it.

Chapter 12

MUSCLES AND JOINTS

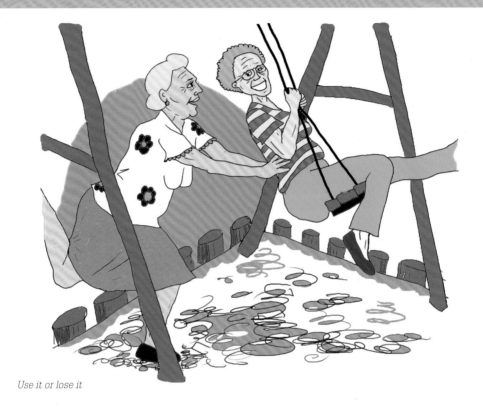

Use it or lose it

Arthritis Research UK reports that there are over 100,000 GP consultations every day in the UK about a musculoskeletal problem. This equates to 21 per cent of us going to see our GP each year about this type of problem. Exercise itself may be to blame for some of these consultations; I'm sure you've all pulled, strained or broken something whilst being active. What's becoming increasingly clear, however, is that exercise is vital in maintaining healthy bones, muscles and joints. Muscle strengthening programmes are just as important for the frail 80-year-old lady trying to avoid a broken hip and maintain her independence as they are for the 20-year-old international bodybuilder. The saying 'use it or lose it' has never been more relevant, and the theory that 'rest is best' when it comes to joints, has been turned on its head. Let's have a closer look at muscles and joints to see why this is the case and what you can do to maximise your musculoskeletal health.

Muscles

There are nearly 700 different muscles in the body, and they fall into three types. First, there's smooth muscle which forms the walls of structures such as your bowel, bladder and blood vessels; you don't have any direct control over smooth muscle. Secondly, there's cardiac muscle, which is only found in the heart. Skeletal muscle is the third type, and it's responsible for movement, so let's look at this type in more detail.

SKELETAL MUSCLE

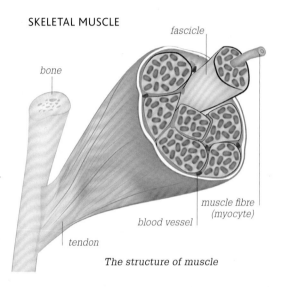

bone

fascicle

muscle fibre
(myocyte)

blood vessel

tendon

The structure of muscle

Muscle cells are called myocytes and in skeletal muscle they form long strands called fibres; they're packed full of mitochondria, which supply energy. The fibres are bundled together in groups called fascicles and blood vessels run in between the fascicles to deliver oxygen to the muscles. The outer layer of muscle forms a tendon, which attaches and firmly anchors the muscle to bone.

There are two types of muscle fibre: type 1, also called slow-twitch and type 2 or fast-twitch. Slow-twitch fibres contract slowly and they take a long time to tire, so they're used for endurance activities like cycling and long distance running. Fast-twitch fibres contract quickly and tire rapidly, so they're designed for explosive movements like jumping and sprinting. How many of each fibre you have is determined by your genetics. Most people will have a 50/50 mix, but the ratio of fast- to slow-twitch fibres may determine which sports you're naturally gifted at. If you have an excess of fast-twitch fibres, you might be joining the Olympic sprinters in the 100 metres. If, however, you have more slow-twitch muscles then a marathon start line might be your destination. It's not clear whether one muscle fibre can be converted into another, but you can certainly train the fibres you do have with the relevant type of activity.

PROBLEMS WITH MUSCLES

Muscle strains and pulls I'm sure you've all pulled or strained a muscle when you've lifted something too heavy or bent awkwardly. When muscle fibres are overstretched, some of them tear. If you get an accompanying bruise, it's because the blood vessels between the fibres have torn too. Thankfully, pulled or strained muscles aren't usually serious and will heal over a few days or weeks. Turn to Chapter 14 to learn how to treat a pulled muscle.

DOMS Have you ever exercised really hard and felt a bit achy and stiff afterwards but then been so sore the next day you can hardly move? This is called DOMS: delayed onset muscle soreness. Muscles hurt and are often stiff, tender and weak. It's common after endurance events, jumping and strength training but any situation where you've really pushed yourself can result in DOMS.

Lactate, also called lactic acid, accumulates in muscles when you exercise hard and used to be blamed for muscle soreness. We now know, however, that lactate levels in the blood return to normal an hour or two after stopping exercise and the muscle soreness in the days afterwards is actually due to tiny tears in the muscle fibres called micro tears. Muscles become inflamed as the body tries to repair them; inflamed, swollen muscles hurt! This discomfort could be your body's way of forcing you to rest and protecting your muscles from further damage while it carries out the repair works.

Warming up and stretching before or after exercising won't prevent DOMS and there are no supplements proven to stop it either. Gradually increasing the intensity or duration of exercise will allow your muscles time to adapt, and is the best way to reduce the likelihood and severity of DOMS. Ice baths might be beneficial too.

DOMS only lasts a few days (usually between three and five). Ice packs, warm baths and painkilling medications can make you feel more comfortable, as can gentle massage and easy exercise. You can return to full activity as soon as you feel able to but it's best to do this gradually.

After my first marathon, my thighs hurt so much I could only navigate the stairs backwards; even gentle walking hurt. I discovered that a 10-minute cold bath, with ice cubes in it, followed by a hot bath really helped speed up my recovery time. Now I'm a more experienced runner I only tend to get DOMS when I do anything that isn't running related. Susie Chan, endurance runner

Cramp Spasms of muscles are caused by a sudden shortening and contraction of the muscle fibres; they're often unexpected and very painful. They usually only last a few minutes, but can have you hopping around and squealing with their intensity. They're more common in pregnancy and with exercise, and they can be a side effect of medications. Sometimes they're just totally spontaneous too. If a muscle is overworked it's easy to understand why it might cramp up in objection but other causes include random nerve stimulation, reduced blood flow and disturbances in the salt balance of the body.

If you get a cramp, you need to stretch the muscle out. How you do this depends on which muscle is cramping, but the calf muscles are the most commonly affected. To ease a calf cramp, you need to stretch down the back of your lower leg. Do this by lying with outstretched legs and using a scarf to pull your foot and toes towards you. Alternatively, stand on a step with your heels hanging off the back of the step and gradually let your body weight push your heels downwards to give a good stretch down the back of your calves. Gently massaging the tense muscle helps, and if these cramps occur frequently then massaging and stretching a few times during the day may prevent them, although the scientific evidence isn't clear as to whether this is beneficial.

See your GP if: you suffer frequent, disabling cramps without an obvious cause.

Restless legs syndrome There's a condition called 'restless leg syndrome' (RLS). Restless legs can ache, itch, hurt, crawl, tingle or jerk and the only thing that eases them is movement. They're worse in the evenings and at night so fidgety, disturbed

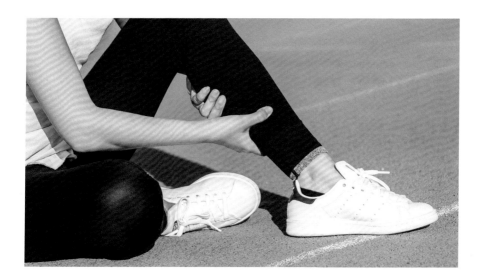

sleep is common. Women are affected twice as often as men and RLS is a common condition in pregnancy. RLS might be a minor inconvenience from time to time or a daily nightmare affecting mood, sleep and quality of life. The cause is unclear but it's felt to be due to a disturbance in neurotransmitters such as dopamine (turn to Chapter 8 to learn more about neurotransmitters). You might develop restless legs if you have other conditions such as hypothyroidism, if you're deficient in iron or as a side effect of certain medications. I've had patients complain that they only experience restless legs after a long session of exercise. Overexertion may be a trigger but in reality there's no clear link for moderate exercise as a cause for RLS and it may actually be beneficial in preventing it, as can cutting out alcohol and caffeine. Medications are reserved for treating severe cases, once underlying causes have been ruled out.

See your GP if: you frequently have restless legs or they're affecting your quality of life.

LOOKING AFTER YOUR MUSCLES

When you consider the demand you place on your muscles, especially when you're exercising regularly, it makes sense that to get the best out of them, you need to look after them. Here are some steps you can take to keep your muscles in top condition.

Warm up well. Whatever type or intensity of exercise you're doing, always warm up your muscles beforehand. This doesn't have to involve a complicated routine and can be as simple as marching on the spot. Ten minutes is an ideal duration for a warm-up. Putting a sudden demand on a cold muscle can cause injuries such as pulled muscles.

Stretching. Don't stand and stretch a cold muscle. Static stretches before exercise won't reduce your risk of injury or muscle soreness; save these stretches for after you've cooled down. If you're keen to do them before you exercise or as an individual stretching session, after a good warm-up is the best time. You can, however, use dynamic stretches before exercise as part of your warm-up. Dynamic stretches involve stretching and moving at the same time and include exercises like arm swings, hip circles, squats and lunges.

Increase load gradually. The key to increasing any activity is to do it in small steps. Muscles need to adapt to change, whether it's the intensity of what you're doing, the duration of your exercise or the number of times a week you do it. Steps which are too big result in muscle fatigue and injury. Follow the '10 per cent rule' and don't increase your efforts by more than this each week. For example, if you've started on a walking programme and walked for a total of 180 minutes during the week, the next step would be to add another 18 minutes to that total the following week. You can apply it to any activity to help you improve steadily, consistently and safely.

THE 10 PER CENT RULE IS ONLY A GUIDE AND YOU MUST ALWAYS LISTEN TO YOUR BODY. SMALLER STEPS OR COMPLETE REST MIGHT BE MORE APPROPRIATE FOR YOU.

Cool down well. Cooling down is often skimped on, but it's just as important as warming up when it comes to caring for your muscles. When you exercise, the blood flow to your muscles increases. If you stop abruptly then that blood can pool in your muscles, particularly your legs, and you can feel faint and dizzy. It's better to slow down gradually and allow your heart rate and muscle contractions to slowly come back to a resting level. During the cool-down, the body will also be eliminating any waste products that have built up in muscle cells during activity. Just five to ten minutes of walking is all that's needed and you can then follow on with some static stretches to your warm pliable muscles.

Recovery. Being lazy is actually good for you; yes, it's official! Muscles need time to adapt to the new stresses you've put on them. In the hours and days following exercise, the microtears in the muscle fibres are repaired, new muscle forms to increase your strength, and energy stores are replenished. How much recovery time you need varies according to your age, health, fitness and the intensity of your exercise session. As a minimum you should have one day a week when you don't exercise, but if you're a beginner or have trained very hard you may need two or even three days' rest. As you get older you need longer for recovery and it's really important to listen to your body to determine when you're ready to exercise again. Gentle activity is fine on recovery days, but avoid anything that puts strain on your adapting muscles.

Eat well. Glucose is the primary energy source for muscle cells. When your glucose levels drop your muscle turns to its stores. Glycogen is the storage form of glucose; it's made up of lots of glucose molecules joined together. It can be released from your liver and muscles, where it's stored, and quickly broken down into individual glucose molecules for use by cells. If you've exercised for over an hour, you need to replenish those glycogen stores. Muscles also need protein to help them repair and recover.

Eating a snack containing a mix of carbohydrate and protein within 30 to 60 minutes of finishing exercise is the optimum way to achieve this. A glass of milk and a handful of brazil nuts is my favourite but other suggestions might be yoghurt and fruit, lentil soup or boiled eggs and toast.

Drink well. It's important to ensure you keep well-hydrated during and after exercise. Water is our ideal fluid replacement but body salts like sodium are lost through our sweat so you need to think about replacing these too if you're sweating excessively in a workout of over 60 to 90 minutes. Muscle cramps and twitching can be triggered by a fall in body salts, so it's sensible to use a sports drink containing electrolytes as your fluid replacement in these situations.

OTHER MUSCLE RECOVERY TECHNIQUES

Massage   When muscles are cramped, tight or sore massage is often used to ease discomfort. This can range from gently rubbing a muscle yourself to a deep tissue massage by a professional. Many people regularly indulge in a sports massage to help ease muscular tension and keep them exercising. Interestingly, it's hard to find scientific evidence to support this practice. Most scientific studies don't show that massage

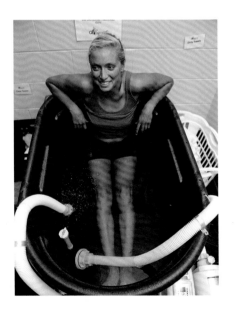

makes any significant improvement to recovery. We certainly don't have clear evidence to suggest which intensity, timing and duration of massage will give the most benefits. There may be a benefit from any psychological pleasure massage brings (although sports massage is often very painful) and anecdotally many people swear that massage helps to keep them active but whether and how it aids muscle recovery and performance is an area that needs more research.

Ice baths   We've all seen the pictures and videos of athletes plunging themselves into ice-cold water baths after exercise; you're braver than me if you've tried it! The theory is that rapidly cooling muscles will reduce inflammation and swelling, prevent DOMS and speed up recovery. Ice baths sway in and out of fashion, but currently there remains fierce debate as to their benefit. A Cochrane review (a systematic review of all the available evidence on a subject) in 2012 concluded that there was some evidence that ice baths reduce DOMS but not enough evidence to make other claims. It may be that by reducing the inflammatory process it interferes with the body's repair mechanism, and that might hinder, rather than help, muscle recovery.

Foam rolling Foam rollers are firm cylinders of various sizes and textures. The idea is to use your own body weight to compress your muscles against the foam. The process is also called myofascial release. 'Myo' means muscle and 'fascia' is the name for the tissue that surrounds muscle. During repetitive exercise, the fascia can thicken and stick to muscles in places, restricting their movement. Myofascial release aims to break up the sticky bits and free up the underlying muscle. It's a hugely popular technique, particularly in those who enjoy endurance sports which involve lots of repetitive movements. Foam rollers are found in most gyms now and seem to be an established part of the fitness world. There are, however, lots of unknowns. How much pressure should you use? How long should you roll for? What's the best rolling technique? Will foam rolling reduce injury risk and improve performance, or just ease sore muscles? These are all unanswered questions and clearly there's a lot of research to be done to determine exactly the best way to use foam rolling for good muscle health.

Compression garments More and more often you'll see people exercising wearing compression garments, or putting them on after exercise to help their recovery. This is yet another area where more research needs to be done before a clear verdict can be given as to whether wearing tight-fitting clothes that stabilise and compress underlying tissues will improve performance, reduce injury or help recovery. At the moment they seem to be most useful as a recovery aid for sore, tired leg muscles, but there's no clear evidence that they'll improve your performance.

Joints

Joints are where bone meets bone, and there are different types of joints in your body determined by the purpose of the joint and the directions it needs to move in. Shoulder and hips are 'ball and socket' joints because they move in all directions. Knee and fingers are hinge joints as they bend and straighten. Some joints aren't designed to move at all, such as the joints linking the bones of our skull. There are several things

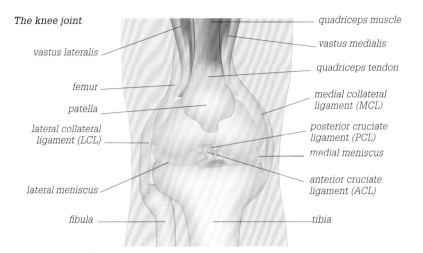

The knee joint

vastus lateralis

femur

patella

lateral collateral
ligament (LCL)

lateral meniscus

fibula

quadriceps muscle

vastus medialis

quadriceps tendon

medial collateral
ligament (MCL)

posterior cruciate
ligament (PCL)

medial meniscus

anterior cruciate
ligament (ACL)

tibia

that the moveable joints have in common:

◎ **Articular cartilage** – a firm coating on the end of bones which provides a smooth surface, preventing bone moving directly against bone and reducing friction.

◎ **Ligaments** – tough fibrous bands which stabilise joints.

◎ **Synovial fluid** – this fluid bathes joints to lubricate them; it's made by the synovial membrane lining the joint cavity.

◎ **Muscles and tendons** – these move the joint and also absorb impact and add stability.

Looking at the knee joint, you can see how these design parts all fit together. When you walk, your knee has to bear a load up to two and a half times your body weight, and when you jump that increases to up to 10 times. The knee joint has to be immensely strong to withstand these forces. The cartilage in the knee includes the articular cartilage on the end of the bones and the lateral and medial menisci, which act as shock absorbers. There are four main ligaments providing side-to-side and backwards and forwards stability. Finally, the joint is surrounded by an array of powerful muscles (three of which are shown above); these attach to the bones by tendons.

Any part of the joint structure can be damaged. Bones can be broken, ligaments can be sprained, cartilage can be torn and muscles pulled. Turn to Chapter 14 to find out more about these problems.

OSTEOARTHRITIS

Osteoarthritis (OA) is the commonest type of arthritis, causing joint pain to an estimated 8.5 million people in the UK and 27 million people in the USA. It usually

Fibromyalgia

Fibromyalgia (FM) is a poorly-understood, long-term health condition that possibly affects as many as one in 25 people; women are affected up to 10 times as often as men. Sufferers of FM have large amounts of pain in various parts of their body or sometimes an all-over body pain usually accompanied by fatigue and sleep disturbance. Muscles and joints feel achy, stiff and swollen and headaches, dizziness and low mood can be a feature too. We don't know what causes it, it can't be cured and the aim of treatment is to ease the pain and disruption that flares of FM cause in everyday life. Treatments include medications to ease pain and help mood, but also behavioural therapies to help people cope with how FM makes them feel. Exercise is emerging as an important strategy in FM treatment. Cochrane reviews of all relevant medical research papers have been carried out in 2007, 2013 and 2014. At each of these reviews they've indicated that there are few large, high-quality studies to draw data from but they've found benefits in exercise. Supervised aerobic training improved symptoms of FM and the overall fitness of the people studied. Moderate- to high-intensity resistance training has potential to improve pain, tenderness, muscle strength and ability to do normal activities. Taking part in aquatic training where exercises are done standing in water may improve symptoms of FM, along with fitness and feelings of wellness. If you have FM and want to use exercise to help your symptoms it needs to be started slowly, increased gradually and ideally supervised by a health professional trained in this specific area.

affects the hips, knees, spine, hands and big toes. We might know it as 'wear and tear' arthritis, but this name is misleading as it insinuates that we've damaged our joints by using them. In fact, the opposite is true: we're more likely to damage our joints by being inactive and not using them.

OA is actually an active process that's repairing joints. It's much more accurate to call it 'wear and repair'. We need our joints to be functioning normally and pain-free so any damage is quickly noted and all parts of the joint work together to repair it. The joint may change in its structure, small areas of cartilage may be lost and bone shape may change, but ultimately these changes are evidence the joint is under active repair.

OA has certain characteristics on an X-ray. However, X-rays are rarely taken to make the diagnosis because they can be misleading. Some people with severe changes on an X-ray may not have any pain from a joint, whereas others who have minimal OA changes on an X-ray can have a lot of discomfort. OA doesn't always progress, either: mild changes may remain static for years. Your doctor will usually make the diagnosis by listening to your symptoms and examining your joint. Affected joints hurt more when you use them and the pain eases when you rest. They can swell a little and their movement can be restricted. After resting, joints can be stiff.

The problem comes when there's a mismatch between the wear and repair. If the wear is excessive, the repair may not be able to keep up, and if the repair processes are slow then a small amount of wear will have a larger effect.

Excessive wear happens if the load you're placing on the joint is more than it was designed for; this is the case if you're overweight. Excessive wear on all or part of a joint also happens if the joint isn't properly aligned, such as when you exercise with an injury or an unbalanced posture. A joint that's been damaged by a previous bone fracture is more at risk of OA because it's likely to be misaligned and there may be too much damage for the repair process to cope with. If you're repeatedly stressing any joint and not allowing enough time for the repair before you stress it again, wear will outpace repair and the joint will be damaged.

The repair process tends to slow as you get older, and this is why you need to allow more time for recovery as you age. Repair may also be inadequate if you're malnourished and your diet doesn't contain essential vitamins and minerals needed for good joint health. OA does seem to run in some families and although a clear genetic link hasn't been identified it's thought that we may inherit multiple genes which make joints more susceptible to breaking down.

Exercise and osteoarthritis We're only now beginning to really understand the power that exercise has in preventing and treating osteoarthritis (OA). Historically, the assumption has been that resting to avoid further joint damage is the best course of action. As a result, people have become very inactive, confirmed by a study published in Arthritis and Rheumatism in 2011 which reported that 57 per cent of women with knee OA in the USA had done no moderate activity of more than 10 minutes during the previous week. This is not only harmful to joints, but also to general health. The fear of wearing out joints or causing more damage in those who already have OA is a major barrier stopping many people exercising, but there's significant evidence that being active will prevent OA developing, improve the function of joints affected by OA and reduce pain caused by it too. A study published in the American Journal of Preventive Medicine in 2008 followed long-distance runners and non-runners over a 20-year period. The runners didn't have any more frequent or severe OA than the non-runners at the end of the study. There are some factors, however, that will increase your risk of OA when you exercise. These include exercising with an injury, poor biomechanics and being overweight. Any increased link with arthritis in footballers' knees is felt to be caused by the larger number of injuries, and similarly the higher BMI of weightlifters could account for the larger numbers affected by knee arthritis. There are tips to minimise your own risk in the 'Looking after your joints' section later on.

ARTHRITIS IS MORE COMMON IN PEOPLE THAT ARE INACTIVE AND OBESE COMPARED TO THOSE THAT EXERCISE REGULARLY.

How to exercise with osteoarthritis

It's important to do both aerobic exercise that gets your heart pumping and resistance exercises to build muscle strength if you have OA. You should still be aiming for the 150 minutes of moderate exercise recommended by the World Health Organisation, but if you have joint pain or haven't exercised before then this may be the goal you aim towards rather than your starting point. Exercise may feel a little uncomfortable at first, but persevere, because over time the muscles and joints will strengthen and pain will reduce. Low-impact exercises like walking or cycling are ideal if you have established and painful OA. Swimming or walking in the pool will provide aerobic exercise with minimal impact on your joints if your condition is severe.

It can be difficult to know how much exercise is too much, and often trial and error will be your guide. Always start slowly and build up gradually. It's normal for a joint to ache afterwards, but if your pain is severe or your joint becomes hot and swollen these are signs that you've done too much. That doesn't mean exercise isn't for you; it just means you need to do a little less next time. Let the joints recover for a day or two and start again at a reduced intensity when they feel comfortable.

Arthritis Research UK have lots of useful information on their website and they've

I'm a PE teacher and I've always enjoyed lots of different sports like hockey, golf and skiing. I had to have a hip replacement because of arthritis; unfortunately the operation was complicated and for a while afterwards I could hardly walk. I had to have hydrotherapy and physio for two years. I was determined to get back to exercising; sport is part of who I am and I needed to regain some of my identity. It's not been easy but it's been worth it and I'm now cycling and swimming. I've entered a 60-mile cycle sportive and a one-mile open water swim. I'm also back sharing my love of exercise with my pupils. Alison Wood, 60, primary school teacher

> YOU CAN BREAK EXERCISE UP INTO 10-MINUTE BLOCKS IF YOU FIND THAT LONGER SESSIONS ARE TOO PAINFUL FOR YOUR JOINTS.

produced a booklet called 'Keep Moving', which focuses on the benefits of exercise in arthritis and details specific strengthening exercises for a range of joints.

See your GP if: your arthritis is causing pain that's interfering with your daily life or making you unable to exercise. There are a range of painkillers that may be beneficial ▪ you have multiple joints which are painful, swollen and tender ▪ any morning stiffness of your joints is lasting more than 30 minutes.

RHEUMATOID ARTHRITIS

Rheumatoid arthritis (RA) is fundamentally different to osteoarthritis. It's what we call an inflammatory arthritis, and it's an auto-immune condition where the body starts to attack itself. In RA it's the joints that are under fire, and the inflammation leads to painful, swollen, tender joints which are ultimately damaged and destroyed by the process. It most commonly affects the small joints of our hands, feet and wrists, but bigger joints can be affected too. Women are three times more likely than men to suffer with RA, but it isn't a common condition with 400,000 people in the UK affected. It can, however, be very destructive and lead to long-term pain and disability. If the condition is picked up early a specialist can prescribe disease-modifying anti-rheumatic drugs (DMARDs) to slow down the damage to joints. Fatigue is also a common complaint with RA, particularly during flare-ups which characterise the condition.

Exercise is important in managing RA and you should take advice from a specialist physiotherapist about the types and intensity of exercise that are suitable for you. Having RA puts you at greater risk of osteoporosis, and muscle mass seems to be lost more quickly too. Strength and resistance exercises will help to minimise bone and muscle loss. Unfortunately, there's a higher risk of heart disease with RA, so cardiovascular exercise is vital; swimming and cycling are ideal if weight bearing causes pain. Exercise will also help you maintain a normal weight, which reduces the stress on your joints and help you to cope with the mental demands that this long-term condition places on you. Movement is often limited by pain, so speak to your GP if your pain is not well-controlled. You need to find the balance between activity and rest that suits you and be prepared to be flexible and adapt your routines during flares.

Looking after your joints

Once you understand more about your joints it becomes easier to see what steps you can take to protect them. Here are some important things you can do to help preserve your joint health.

◎ **Maintain a normal weight.** Reduce the load you place on your joints by losing weight if you need to.
◎ **Train sensibly.** Gradually increasing the intensity, duration and frequency of your exercise will allow all the structures in and around your joints to adapt to the increased work being demanded of them. If you're running, switching from concrete to softer terrain like grass or trails will reduce the impact on your joints.
◎ **Ensure adequate recovery.** Make sure you schedule rest days and lighter activities after strenuous exercise for the natural repair processes to take place; this is particularly important as you grow older.
◎ **Maintain good biomechanics.** Don't exercise when injured as your normal joint alignment is disrupted. If you have any concerns about your posture or you want to train seriously for a big physical challenge, having a check over by a physiotherapist can help to spot any issues before problems arise. If they analyse your gait they can also advise on the correct type of footwear.
◎ **Build muscle strength.** Strengthening and conditioning your muscles is essential for preserving your joints. Strong muscles around a joint will take the strain and impact off a joint so there's less wear to repair. Strength work also stimulates bone production and stronger muscles help to prevent injury too. Get some advice from a personal trainer to get a personalised exercise plan.
◎ **Eat well.** The exact link between diet and joint health isn't fully established but eating a healthy, varied diet rich in vitamins and minerals will ensure your body has all the building blocks needed for healthy joints. It's important to include calcium-rich foods such as dairy products and omega-3 fatty acids, which can be found in oily fish. There's fierce debate when it comes to the benefit of nutritional supplements. There's no supplement that will slow down the progression of arthritis. Omega-3 fatty acids can help reduce pain in an inflammatory arthritis like rheumatoid arthritis, but not osteoarthritis. Glucosamine sulphate may help to reduce pain from osteoarthritis of the knee, but at present there's not enough evidence to recommend it.

Chapter 13

COMMON ILLNESSES

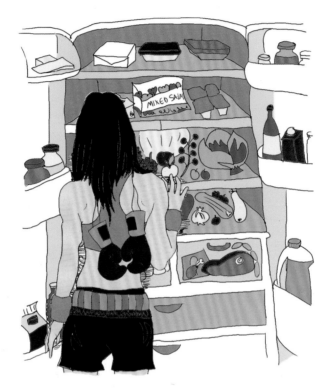

*Fuel well
for health*

Exercising regularly keeps you fit and healthy and you'll find you're ill less often than your sedentary friends and colleagues. You'll have more energy at home and work and be more productive and less likely to take sick days. However, there's no escaping the odd germ and all of us will from time to time become unwell. On those days, when getting out of bed is an impossibility, it's obvious we can't exercise. Sometimes, however, the decision can be a little less black and white. It can be hard to know whether you're well enough, whether it'll make you worse or speed up your recovery. It's very tempting to push on with your planned session, when in fact, you'd be better staying under the duvet. There's a fine balance to be struck: overexertion can lead to illness and injury. Let's have a look at how the immune system works, some of the common illnesses that might trip you up and how you can achieve a good balance.

The immune system

The body has many mechanisms to keep germs out, from the tiny hairs in your nostrils trapping dust and germs to the acid in your stomach, killing bugs in your food. Despite this, sometimes the front line of defence is broken and your body has to quickly mobilise its troops.

It's your white blood cells that spring into action when a germ invades. White blood cells only make up one per cent of your total blood volume, but they have a vital role in keeping you healthy. There are lots different types of white blood cells including neutrophils, eosinophils, basophils, lymphocytes and monocytes. Between them they have a range of ammunition they can use against invading germs. Some of them produce chemicals which neutralise the toxins that the germ has released. Others literally swallow up the germ and digest it. Lymphocytes carry antibodies which match up to markers called antigens on the surface of germs. Once a match is made the lymphocytes multiply and make lots of copies of the antibody which destroy the germ. This means that if you meet that germ again, your body recognises the antigen and can mount an immediate response.

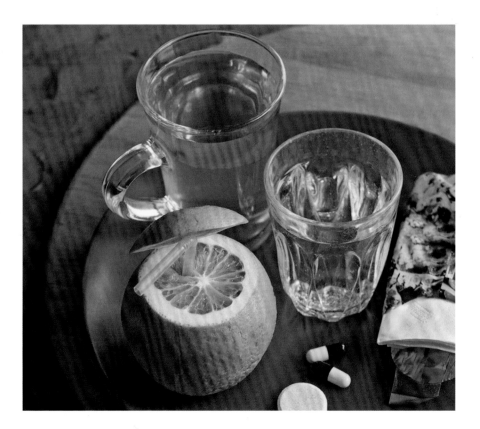

You might get a high temperature (fever) when you have an infection. We don't fully understand the role that a fever has, but we think it makes the environment unfavourable for bacteria and viruses to reproduce. It also seems to support the immune response by triggering the multiplication of white blood cells and antibodies and helping damaged cells to repair themselves. This opens up the question as to whether you should lower a fever while you have an infection, and the answer is unclear. If you don't feel uncomfortable with a fever, then there's probably no need to treat it.

You'll also notice that your heart rate is faster than usual when you're unwell. This is because the energy requirements of your body are higher when you have an infection. To meet those increased demands your heart has to pump blood more quickly around the body. This helpfully speeds up the delivery of the white blood cells to sites of infection too.

Common infections

When you have an active infection your body is concentrating its efforts on fighting it and returning you to health. These processes consume a large proportion of your energy and it's easy to see why your body might not be able to find the extra needed for exercise. To help in the dilemma of whether you should exercise or not, here's a handy checklist for some common, everyday infections.

COMMON COLD

◎   OK to exercise: you've just got a bit of a runny nose and a few sneezes and sniffles, but all your symptoms are above your neck and you don't have a high temperature.

◎   Give it a miss: you've got a high temperature, you feel shivery or achy, your nose is permanently streaming or you're needing to take regular paracetamol to keep your symptoms under control.

SINUS INFECTION

◎   OK to exercise: your sinuses feel a bit congested or tender but you can breathe freely and feel fine in yourself.

◎   Give it a miss: your temperature is high, you feel dizzy or lightheaded, your nasal discharge is very thick and your face or teeth are hurting.

COUGH

◎   OK to exercise: you're coughing occasionally and it's a dry tickly cough that's caused by throat irritation without a high temperature.

◎   Give it a miss: you have a chesty cough with phlegm, you feel out of breath or wheezy when you're walking about or you have a high temperature.

SORE THROAT

◎ OK to exercise: your throat is a bit dry or scratchy but you feel fine in yourself and you can swallow normally.

WE SHOULD ALWAYS LISTEN TO OUR BODY; IT'S RARELY WRONG.

◎ Give it a miss: it's really painful to swallow, you have glands up in your neck making it feel stiff, your temperature is high or you feel shivery.

UPSET STOMACH

◎ OK to exercise: you've only had one small episode of diarrhoea, you feel fine and don't have any stomach cramps or vomiting. You've eaten and drunk something without complication.

◎ Give it a miss: you've had more than one bout of diarrhoea, have stomach cramps, vomiting, nausea or a high temperature.

URINARY INFECTION

◎ OK to exercise: you've had a couple of extra trips to the toilet for a wee and it felt a bit uncomfortable but you're otherwise all right and don't have any abdominal pain or a high temperature.

◎ Give it a miss: it's stinging when you wee, there's blood in your urine or you've got abdominal pain, low back pain or nausea.

Regular exercise definitely helps me stay well. I exercise at least four times a week and only get ill a couple of times a year. I'm careful to make sure I rest enough, especially if I've really pushed myself. If I start to feel generally tired, I know I'm overdoing it and I cut back a bit. Tamsin Threlfall, mum of two, baker (and eater) of cakes

Exercising with an infection

It can be very frustrating to be ill when you're full of motivation and in the swing of a regular exercise plan. The quickest way to get back on your feet is to allow your body to rest for a few days and focus on getting better. Pushing on and stubbornly refusing to take time out will make you feel worse and prolong your illness by dampening your immune response. As mentioned, your heart rate is often faster when you have an infection, particularly if you have a high temperature or you're a bit dehydrated, which is often the case when you're unwell. Pushing your heart rate up further by exercising vigorously can take it to dangerous levels, making you feel dizzy and faint or inducing a harmful irregularity in the rhythm. If you're keen to keep moving and you feel up to it then reduce the intensity of your exercise. Gentle activity like walking is fine and might actually be beneficial in the early stages of a cold. Starting with a short distance and seeing how you feel is the safest way to approach it, and remember to drink plenty of fluids along the way. What's crucial is to listen to your body, be flexible with your plans and remember that it'll take more than a few days for you to lose fitness. Sometimes rest is best.

I was overtraining and developed extreme fatigue. I've come back from this and learnt the hard way that the most important thing is to listen to my body. I make sure I have enough rest days and easier weeks. I have to eat well before and after training and ensure I consume enough calories to fuel my training. I'm now following a bespoke training plan and, with the help of a coach, I'm hoping to qualify for a GB age group spot in duathlon. Beatrice Schaer, 43, running coach and sports therapist

Overtraining

It's possible to have too much of a good thing. If you're training too hard you can feel a bit run-down and tired. You might stop making progress in your fitness and performance, but a good rest and readjustment of your training load will usually sort you out. There's a condition called 'Overtraining Syndrome' (OTS) which is many steps

Protect your immune system

Did you know that after high-intensity exercise and sessions lasting over 90 minutes, your immune system is suppressed for 24 hours? This makes you more likely to pick up infections like coughs and colds. If you find you're always ill it's worth moving your toughest training to a different day of the week. Cramming on a busy commuter train or being around snotty children the morning after a hard workout isn't ideal, although it's often unavoidable.

Tips for keeping well

So, we've learnt that to stay well we need to exercise regularly but also that exercise itself causes stress to the body and too much of that can make us unwell. So, how do you find that balance, and what things can you do to keep active and well? Here are my top tips.

- ◎ **Sleep.** During sleep your body regenerates and restores itself. It's essential, although I appreciate it's often hard to come by for many reasons. Remember, if you're increasing your exercise, your sleep needs to increase too. Going to bed 30 minutes earlier may be all that's needed to top up your energy levels.
- ◎ **Train well.** This just means being sensible and increasing what you do gradually. Whether it's the duration, frequency or intensity of your exercise, small steps are best to allow your body to adapt.
- ◎ **Rest enough.** Rest is as important as exercise. To stay well you need to schedule rest days into your week, especially if you're following a progressive exercise plan.
- ◎ **Respect illness.** Ploughing on through illness will only prolong it. Always return to exercise slowly after illness and be guided by how you feel.
- ◎ **Eat well.** You can't expect your immune system to remain in top condition if you don't fuel it properly. 'Eating a rainbow' by ensuring you have a variety of colours in the fruit and vegetables you consume is a great way to get the vitamins and nutrients needed for good immune health.
- ◎ **Avoid germs.** Easier said than done, but don't forget simple hand-washing; it can reduce the spread of respiratory infections like colds by 20 per cent.
- ◎ **Consider the bigger picture.** Work, family, stress; they all take their toll on your health and immune system. Exercise can help you cope with all of these issues, but you need to look for balance in all areas of your life to keep well.

up from this natural fatigue. True OTS is very rare and it's most common in athletes. The body is quite simply stretched beyond the capability that it has for recovery. Sufferers can be depressed and irritable, have difficulty sleeping, concentrating and motivating themselves. There can be changes in pulse and blood pressure too. Despite weeks or months of rest, performance doesn't pick up. Recovery is possible with a very gradual return to training but for some competitive athletes it can be the end of their career. This shows how fine the balance between exercise and rest can be.

Chapter 14

COMMON INJURIES

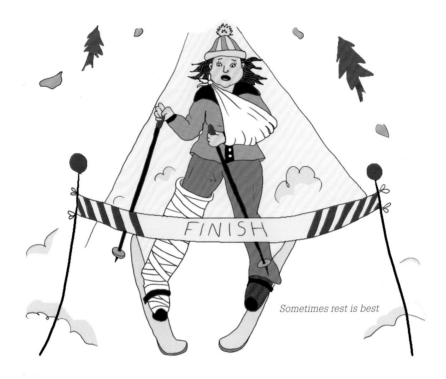

Sometimes rest is best

We all get injured at some point and it can be incredibly frustrating. Spotting and treating injuries early will get you back on track more quickly and prevent any long-term damage. It can be hard to make your own diagnosis and it's always best to get properly assessed by a professional if you think you have more than a minor muscle strain. There are a number of health professionals who can help, including GPs, physiotherapists and podiatrists (experts in conditions of the feet and lower limb), but in some situations you need to go to a minor injuries unit or Accident and Emergency.

When to go to Accident and Emergency

It's tempting to rush off to A&E as soon as you injure yourself but it's not always necessary. Here are some of the scenarios you might find yourself in that do require a trip to the A&E department:

◎ You suspect a broken bone; it might look bent or hurt a lot when you press it.

- You can't weight-bear on a leg or use an arm due to pain.
- You think one of your joints has dislocated (popped out of joint), for example, a shoulder or finger.
- A joint has swollen up suddenly within a few minutes of injuring it.
- You've had a head injury where you've lost consciousness or have any of the warning signs discussed later.

IF FIRST AID ISN'T HELPING AFTER 48–72 HOURS OR IF SYMPTOMS ARE GETTING WORSE YOU NEED TO BE ASSESSED BY A GP OR PHYSIO. IF YOU SUSPECT A BROKEN BONE, GO TO A&E.

If you aren't immediately sure how bad your injury is, use first aid (see the sections on PRICE and painkillers below) and allow some time to see if your symptoms are improving.

The PRICE technique

Use **PRICE** as immediate first aid for any injury to ease pain and promote healing.

Protect stop any further injury occurring.

Rest take weight off and avoid using the injured area.

Ice apply ice for 15 minutes at a time every two hours to ease pain and reduce swelling and inflammation.

Compress use a bandage, such as a tubular elasticated one, to gently squeeze the area and prevent swelling.

Elevate Stop swelling in the injured area by using gravity to drain fluid out of it. Pop your arm in a sling or get your foot up above the level of your hip.

Painkillers

The PRICE technique will help to ease pain, but sometimes painkillers are needed too. Paracetamol should be your first choice; take it regularly (2x500mg tablets every 4–6 hours) for a few days rather than letting the pain build up. The other alternative is NSAIDs (non-steroidal anti-inflammatory drugs) such as ibuprofen. There is, however, a growing body of evidence to suggest that although NSAIDs will reduce pain, they may also slow down healing by dampening the inflammatory reaction that the body is

Hot or cold?

Should we reach for the ice or the hot water bottle when we're injured? For the first 72 hours, cold is best. Use a specially designed ice pack or simply wrap a towel around a bag of frozen peas. Don't put ice directly onto skin as it can cause burns. Apply it for 15 minutes every two hours. Heat should be avoided for the first three days as it increases bleeding, swelling and inflammation. Avoid massage during this time too. Beyond that time both heat and massage are very useful ways to soothe pain. I've seen numerous skin burns from over-zealous heating of injuries so stick with a warm hot water bottle or a wheat bag which can be heated in the microwave.

intentionally provoking to promote repair. If paracetamol and PRICE make you comfortable, avoid NSAIDs for the first 48 hours after an injury. If you have asthma, heartburn or stomach ulcers you may not be able to take NSAIDs so check with a pharmacist. Never take NSAIDs when you're pregnant. NSAIDs such as ibuprofen and diclofenac also come as a cream or gel, these don't always give as much pain relief as the tablet formulas but many people prefer them and there's less chance of side effects.

If these measures haven't eased your pain, you can buy small doses of codeine over the counter. It's sold in combination with paracetamol so make sure you aren't exceeding your maximum dose of paracetamol, which is 4g in 24 hours. If you need to step up to this type of strong medication, you should really be having your injury assessed by a doctor.

SPRAINS AND STRAINS

What: Sprains are overstretched ligaments. Pulled muscles and tendons are known as strains. Some of the most frequently injured include ankles, wrists, groins and hamstrings (muscles at the back of the thigh). The area swells, becomes painful to move, tender and it often bruises.

How: You're more likely to get a strain or sprain if you haven't warmed up properly or if you've had inadequate time to recover from previous exercise. Trying a new type of exercise, overuse or using more force or intensity than usual can also cause them. Sometimes it's a plain old accident but if you have poor stability then twisting and turning leads to wobbling and overstretched muscles and ligaments.

Action: Use the PRICE technique as soon as possible after the injury. After two or three days, when the pain is easing, start stretching and gently moving the injured area. Build up to normal activities gradually and only return to sport once fully healed.

Recovery: Minor strains may heal in a few days. Severe strains and sprains will take several weeks to heal and it can be two to three months before you're ready for sport.

LEG INJURIES

ILIOTIBIAL BAND SYNDROME (ITBS)

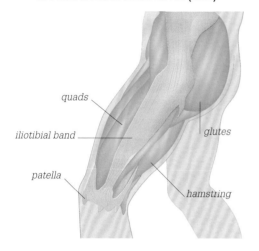

quads

iliotibial band

glutes

patella

hamstring

The iliotibial band

What: The ITB is a band of fibrous tissue that runs from the hip down the outside of the thigh and attaches just below the knee. It helps to stabilise both the hip and knee joints and causes a stabbing pain on the outside of the knee if it's injured. ITBS is linked to underlying biomechanical and postural issues such as muscle weaknesses and the positioning of your knee and foot when you move.

How: ITBS commonly affects runners and cyclists but also rowers, skiers, footballers and weightlifters. It's usually triggered by the friction from suddenly increasing the distance you cover in training.

Action: Cutting back your activity or trying a different one is the first step. A physio assessment will check for underlying postural problems and muscle weaknesses. Strengthening your glutes (bottom muscles) and quads (thigh muscles) is usually advised. Whether stretching the ITB helps is controversial, with some studies suggesting it makes the problem worse. There's similar controversy about deep-massage methods like foam rolling too but it's reasonable to use these techniques alongside ice and anti-inflammatories to see if they ease discomfort.

Recovery: Mild ITBS caught and corrected early can settle in days but more stubborn cases take weeks.

SHIN SPLINTS

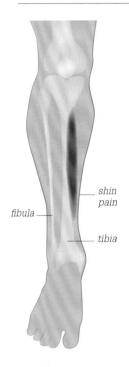

shin pain

fibula

tibia

What: Also known as medial tibial stress syndrome (MTSS). This causes pain on the lower, inside part of the shin bone. Initially it eases soon after stopping exercise, but can progress to hurting at rest. The periosteum, the surface of the bone, becomes inflamed and tender as it's constantly trying to repair the stress that repetitive activity is placing on it. If you have severe pain or tenderness, pain at rest or at night then you need an X-ray to rule out a bone problem like a stress fracture.

How: Most common in runners, but also affects footballers, dancers and basketball players. Increasing training distance, running on hard or uneven surfaces, inappropriate footwear, postural imbalances and biomechanical issues can all cause MTSS.

Action: Use PRICE. Mild MTSS will improve quickly with rest, correction of any underlying issues (see a physio or podiatrist to check for these), and a gradual return to activity.

Recovery: Two to six weeks' rest is required, or longer if a stress fracture is present.

HIP INJURY

TROCHANTERIC BURSITIS

What: Also called greater trochanteric pain syndrome. Pain is felt over the trochanter (the bony prominence at the side of your hip) where tendons insert into the bone; it can be felt deep in the hip and outer thigh too. Friction and sometimes swelling of the bursa (fluid-filled sacs which cushion the area) mean it's painful to touch. It hurts to lie on your side, cross your legs and is worse when you exercise or climb stairs.

How: Women are more at risk than men and it peaks age 40 to 50. It's common in runners and cyclists due to the repetitive movements, or if you've suddenly increased your training load, especially if this involves lots of steps uphill.

Action: Rest and reduced exercise is critical to allow the area to heal. Be guided by pain; if it hurts, you shouldn't be doing it. Ice packs, anti-inflammatories and sometimes steroid injections into the hip will ease discomfort. It's advisable to see a physio to help correct underlying postural problems.

Recovery: Three months or longer.

KNEE INJURIES

KNEE LIGAMENT INJURY

What: There are four main ligaments stabilising the knee joint (turn back to Chapter 12 for a diagram). The collateral ligaments prevent too much side-to-side movement of the knee and the cruciate ligaments provide forwards and backwards stability. These ligaments can get overstretched (sprained) and partially or fully torn (ruptured). You'll get sudden pain, tenderness and either immediate or gradual swelling of your knee and may be unable to weight bear or freely move your knee, which may feel as if it's giving way underneath you.

How: Knee ligaments, particularly the anterior cruciate ligament (ACL) are often damaged during contact sports like football and rugby and during tennis and skiing when you land or fall awkwardly. It's not clear why but ACL injuries are more common in women than men.

Action: Follow the PRICE instructions previously for first aid but suspected ligament injuries should be checked by a doctor. With severe injuries, you might need to wear a knee brace and surgery may be needed at a later date for more complicated injuries, particularly of the cruciate ligaments.

Recovery: Eight to 12 weeks for sprains and six to nine months for ruptures.

KNEE CARTILAGE INJURY

What: The medial (inside) and lateral (outside) menisci are the shock-absorbing cartilage pads in the knee. They can tear part or all of the way across, often at the same time as a ligament strain or rupture. If the tear is small, you might not have many symptoms, but a larger tear makes the knee swell and it can hurt to walk and straighten your leg. Occasionally a fragment of cartilage can get jammed in the joint and the knee locks in a bent position. You might feel a clicking or clunking as the fragment moves.

How: Cartilage injuries are usually due to twisting and turning on a leg that you've already got your weight on so they're common in football, rugby and tennis.

Action: Follow the PRICE instructions. Small tears may heal up themselves but larger tears require surgery, so if your pain isn't settling or your knee movement is affected see your GP for a referral to an orthopaedic specialist. Physiotherapy is ideal to strengthen up the muscles around the knee.

Recovery: Six weeks for a small tear but around eight weeks if surgery is required.

FOOT INJURIES

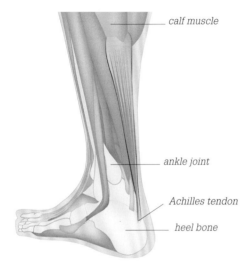

calf muscle

ankle joint

Achilles tendon

heel bone

ACHILLES TENDINOPATHY

What: The Achilles is the thick, strong tendon that connects the calf muscles to the heel. When injured it hurts up the back of the heel at the beginning and end of a training session. If untreated it progresses to constant pain and tendon rupture. Previously called Achilles tendinitis because it was thought to be inflammation (-itis) of the tendon, we now think the actual fibres of the tendon become damaged too.

How: Caused by excessive stress on the tendon during running, especially fast or uphill. It hurts more walking on tip toes or squatting.

Action: Seek help early with Achilles problems; they're easier and quicker to treat in the early stages. Movement is OK if it's pain-free. Use ice packs after exercise. Don't rest completely, stimulate tendon repair by stretching and gently loading the tendon. Rise on your toes and slowly lower down and also perform this movement lowering your heels off the edge of a step; progress to doing it standing on one leg. Calf massage, heel inserts and sports taping are other techniques that may help; see a physio for advice.

Recovery: Two weeks to six months; if lasting beyond this it may need surgery.

PLANTAR FASCIITIS (PF)

What: PF is inflammation of the tissues of the sole of the foot. It's usually felt as pain in your heel when you walk, especially when getting out of bed in the morning or after a day on your feet. The pain can spread up the outside of your foot towards your ankle. It can affect one or both feet and it can be extremely painful.

How: This is common in endurance sports such as long-distance running but anyone who's on their feet a lot can be affected and it's more common if you wear unsupportive shoes such as ballet pumps.

Action: Rest until the pain eases. Anti-inflammatory painkillers and ice packs can ease the discomfort. Try rolling a tennis ball or a bottle of frozen water under the foot to massage it. Put a scarf under the ball of your foot and pull the ends towards you to stretch the underside of your foot. Gel heel pads in good supportive shoes can ease pain, and try wearing a shoe with a heel to move the pressure onto the toes. Avoid walking barefoot.

Recovery: Two weeks to six months, occasionally up to 12 months.

SHOULDER INJURY

ROTATOR CUFF INJURIES

What: The rotator cuff is the name given to the four muscles which encircle the shoulder joint. These muscles are anchored into the shoulder bone by a large tendon. This tendon can get pinched and rub against the collar bone; this is called impingement. It causes pain in and around the shoulder, often down the arm and is worse when you lift your arm above your head. The rotator cuff can also tear, partially or fully, leading to pain, muscle weakness and restricted movement of the shoulder.

How: Shoulder injuries can happen gradually with overuse or suddenly after an accident like a fall. Repetitive and intensive training, particularly where your arm is overhead such as in tennis, swimming, weightlifting and throwing, are high risk for shoulder injuries.

Action: Avoid activities that hurt and use ice and painkillers for discomfort. Don't rest it completely; regular gentle movement of the shoulder will stop it stiffening up. Seek advice from a GP or physio if it's not improving after three days, or sooner if pain is uncontrolled. Steroid injections into the shoulder may be an option and sometimes surgery is required.

Recovery: Two to six weeks for impingement and four to six months after rotator cuff surgery.

ELBOW INJURY

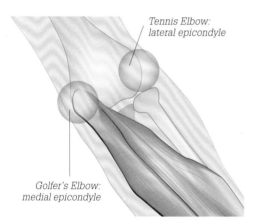

Tennis Elbow: lateral epicondyle

Golfer's Elbow: medial epicondyle

TENNIS ELBOW AND GOLFER'S ELBOW

What: Your epicondyles are the prominent bones on either side of your elbow. Damage to the tendons which attach at these points causes pain around the elbow and in the forearm, especially when gripping, lifting and twisting things. Symptoms around the outside (lateral) epicondyle are called tennis elbow. Golfer's elbow affects the inside (medial) epicondyle.

How: It's commonest age 40 to 50, and is due to strenuous repetitive movements. Tennis and other racquet sports can cause it, as can throwing sports like the javelin, but more often it's triggered by simple activities at home like gardening or decorating.

Action: Avoid activities that cause pain and use ice and painkillers like ibuprofen to ease discomfort. Using a lighter racquet with a bigger grip size and changing your technique can help if racquet sports have been the trigger. Injections of steroid, physiotherapy and occasionally surgical treatments might be required for stubborn cases.

Recovery: Usually resolves within a year.

BACK PAIN AND SCIATICA

What: Most people get back pain at some point in their lives. You can strain or sprain the muscles and ligaments in your back and arthritis can sometimes affect the spinal joints, but often there isn't any cause and it's called 'non-specific back pain'. Nerves can

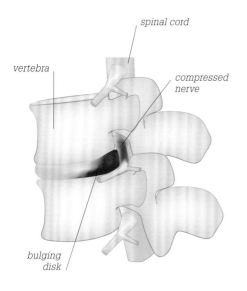

spinal cord

vertebra

compressed nerve

bulging disk

Sciatica

get trapped on their journey from the spine to your muscles and compressing a nerve causes pain, tingling or numbness along its course. The sciatic nerve is commonly affected, especially in pregnancy. It travels from your lower back, through your buttocks and down the back of your legs. When it's compressed and causing symptoms it's called sciatica. It usually gets squashed by a 'slipped disc'. Discs are gel-filled pads between each of the vertebrae (spine bones); they don't actually slip, but their contents can bulge, prolapse and press on nerves.

How: Sudden movements, falls or lifting a heavy weight can injure your back, as can poor posture, but back pain can also happen spontaneously without an obvious cause.

Action: It's far better to keep moving about gently and use painkillers, hot and cold compresses and stretching to enable you to return to your usual activities and job as soon as possible. There are examples of stretches to ease low back pain at www.nhs.uk. If the pain isn't settling within six weeks, see your GP who may arrange some tests or refer you to a physiotherapist.

Recovery: One to six weeks for simple back pain. Keeping generally fit and active will help to prevent recurrence.

HEAD INJURIES

What: Minor bangs to the head can give you a headache and make you feel sick and dizzy, but severe injuries can cause devastating brain damage. The term 'concussion' refers to head injuries where someone's lost consciousness for a few minutes, had memory loss, blurred vision or been briefly confused but otherwise made a full recovery.

How: Falls, clashes of heads and collisions with cars whilst cycling or running can all cause exercise-related head injuries. Skull bones are protective, but your brain can move a little inside your skull and damage occurs as it gets shaken around.

Action: You need to go immediately to A&E if you have any signs that suggest a more serious brain injury, including any loss of consciousness, drowsiness, any indication of a skull fracture such as obvious injury or clear fluid or blood coming from the nose or ears, a seizure (fit), blurred or double vision, vomiting, memory loss, difficulties with speaking, reading or writing, weakness or inability to walk, persistent headache, confusion, unusual behaviour or if you take anticoagulants (blood thinning medication). If you have a minor head injury, ask someone to stay with you for 24 hours. If you develop any of the above symptoms go to A&E. Otherwise, rest, use a cold compress on the injured area and take paracetamol for pain.

Recovery: A few days for a minor bump. You can return to exercise when you feel well enough, but avoid contact sports for three weeks.

Keeping fit whilst injured

Being injured doesn't mean you can't do any exercise. It can actually be a time when you increase your strength and endurance. You just need to be flexible and imaginative. If you can't do weight-bearing exercise you can often still swim. If you've injured your arm, a static bike can become your new best friend. Sometimes you'll discover a new sport that you love, and cross-training (using a sport other than your regular one) is a great way to work different muscle groups and generally improve your strength and fitness. Using your injury time to work on improving your core strength will help to prevent further injuries when you return to full activity. Try to remain positive and look on injury as an opportunity to learn about your body.

Returning to exercise after an injury

Obviously the best way to return to activity after an injury is to do it gradually. You can't just pick up where you left off. This might mean starting with short, gentle walks to ease yourself in gently over a number of weeks. What's crucial is that you take time to consider why you got injured in the first place. Perhaps it was a simple accident like a fall, but often the underlying cause is a muscle imbalance or weakness. If you haven't taken any steps to correct these issues, re-injury is very likely. Ideally get checked by a physiotherapist or a podiatrist (for foot or leg problems) to spot such issues before you return to activity. You can then work on specific exercises to strengthen muscles and stabilise joints. A gait analysis to ensure you're wearing the correct shoes is helpful; this involves running on a treadmill whilst being filmed so your foot positioning can be observed. Many stores selling sports shoes offer a gait analysis and having the right shoes may reduce your injury risk.

It's always a good idea to tell any instructors or coaches that you're returning from injury so they can advise you whether there are any specific exercises you should avoid. If you've had an injury like plantar fasciitis or sciatica where high impact has been part of the cause, try exercising on a softer terrain like grass or a treadmill for some or all of your sessions to reduce impact. Turn back to Chapter 12 for advice on how to look after your muscles and joints to prevent injury.

It takes discipline and patience to make an effective return to exercise after injury. You should be completely pain-free before you start, take it frustratingly slowly and listen to your body.

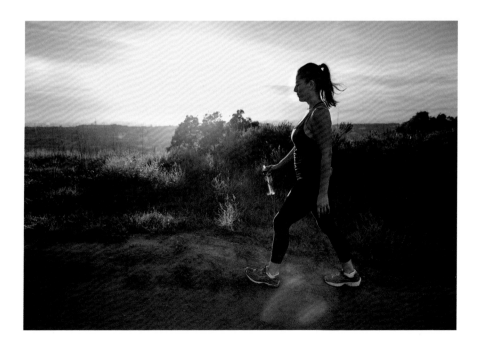

Chapter 15

COMMON MEDICAL PROBLEMS

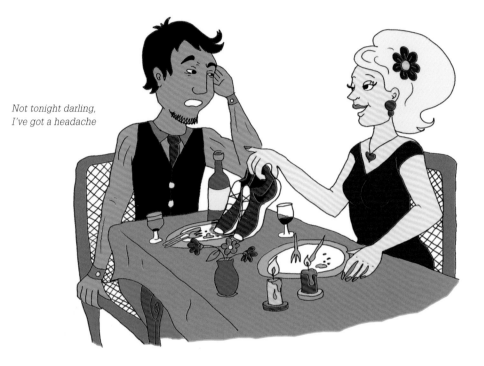

*Not tonight darling,
I've got a headache*

Let's consider some of the common medical problems that we face when trying to keep exercising. What can seem a trivial issue or niggle can turn into a reason not to exercise; our body doesn't always make it easy for us! With a bit of knowledge and a few tricks of the trade most problems can be sorted, leaving us free to enjoy ourselves. This is by no means an exhaustive list but these are the things that crop up the most in my day-to-day work.

Rhinitis

Rhinitis might not be a term you're familiar with, but it's something you've most certainly experienced. It comes from the Greek words *rhin* meaning nose and *itis* meaning inflammation. Rhinitis is characterised by sneezing and a runny or blocked nose. If you're unlucky you might also have itching, inflammation of your eyes (conjunctivitis) or inflamed sinuses (sinusitis).

There are many types of rhinitis. Infective rhinitis is usually caused by a virus and is better known as the common cold. Allergic rhinitis includes allergies to pets, dust mites and pollen. If pollen causes it, it's called hay fever, which affects one in five people in the UK. Sometimes rhinitis can be due to an irritant like dust or chemicals. Swimming in chlorinated pools can make you sneeze and some ski gloves come with a built-in absorbable pad to wipe nose drips triggered by cold mountain air! When you exercise your body cleverly opens up your nasal

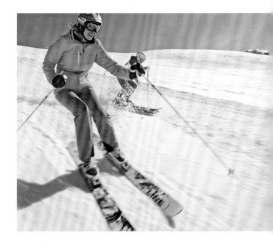

passages as much as possible to allow maximum air flow but this means more exposure to nasal irritants. Sometimes, rhinitis can happen whether you exercise inside or out, regardless of other triggers or allergies and this is called exercise-induced rhinitis. It's more common during long exercise sessions and more severe if you suffer from nasal allergies. It can be very frustrating, inconvenient and can affect your performance.

EXERCISING WITH HAY FEVER

The hay fever season can be a long one, depending on which pollens you're sensitive to. Tree pollens can be released as early as February and grass pollens from May to July, but if you're allergic to weeds and moulds you might suffer right through until October. This can make exercising pretty tricky but if you Count, Cover and Clean you'll limit your contact with pollens as much as possible:

Count. In the UK the Met Office produces a daily pollen forecast so you can avoid exercising outdoors when the count is at its highest. Pollen counts are lower during and after rain and on cooler, still days.

Cover. Wrap-around sunglasses will help prevent pollen getting into your eyes. A light scarf covering your nose and mouth and a hat with a brim will reduce the pollen reaching your face and a dab of Vaseline just inside your nose can stop pollen entering.

Clean. After exercising outside, showering, washing your hair and changing your clothes will minimise your contact with pollen. It's best to dry the clothes indoors rather than outdoors where they'll pick up more pollen. Try using a saline (salt water) nasal wash to remove pollen from the nose.

MEDICATIONS FOR ALLERGIC RHINITIS

Despite your best efforts to avoid contact with allergic triggers (allergens) you can still be badly affected by nasal symptoms. A pharmacy is the first place to go for advice about medications because the majority of treatments for allergic rhinitis are available to buy over the counter.

Antihistamines. Mast cells are present in the lining of nasal passages; they contain histamine, which they release when they come into contact with an allergen; this starts your allergic reaction. Antihistamines block the effects of histamine, which lessens the reaction. An antihistamine tablet will work throughout your body or you can target the antihistamine to your eyes, using eye drops, or your nose via a nasal spray. Look for an antihistamine tablet which is taken once a day for convenience. Most are 'non-sedating' which means they shouldn't make you drowsy. It's safe to use the tablets every day and if one brand doesn't work, it's worth trying a different one.

Steroids. Steroids help to dampen down inflammation. Due to their side effects, steroid tablets are reserved for severe, uncontrolled allergic reactions. Nasal sprays containing steroids are very helpful in managing the annoying nasal symptoms of allergic rhinitis. They need to be used every day to be effective and can take a week or two to work, so be patient! It's safe to use them alongside antihistamines.

Others. Some medications try to stop the mast cells releasing the histamine in the first place. Eye drops and nasal sprays containing drugs like sodium cromoglicate do this, but like steroids, they need to be taken regularly to be effective. Very blocked noses can be eased with decongestant sprays or tablets but you should only use these for a few days at a time. Another option for very watery, runny noses is a nasal spray containing

Any time I go for a run my nose starts dripping, which is frustrating as I always have to carry hankies. I never have the problem with any indoor exercise. Allergy season makes it even worse and I have to rely on antihistamines. Fiona, fitness fanatic ipratropium; this needs to be prescribed by a doctor. It won't help a blocked nose but may help a runny nose induced by exercise.

See your GP if: your allergic rhinitis is not controlled by medications from your pharmacy. Prescription medication or specialist treatment may be required.

Raynaud's disease

You expect cold fingers and toes if you're outside on a chilly day, but there's a condition called Raynaud's disease which takes this to the extreme. According to Scleroderma and Raynaud's UK, it affects 10 million people in the UK and it's more common in women than men. The small blood vessels in fingers (and less commonly, toes, ears and noses) become extremely sensitive to temperature and constrict (close up) on exposure to the cold. Emotional stress and hormonal changes can be triggers too. Your fingers turn white, numb and eventually blue as the blood supply reduces. When your fingers warm up they flush bright red as the blood vessels open up again and this process can be extremely painful.

In less than 10 per cent of people, Raynaud's is due to an underlying medical condition such as scleroderma or rheumatoid arthritis. For the remaining 90 per cent, there's no cause and treatment focuses on trying to avoid your extremities getting cold. This can be tricky if you want to exercise outdoors, so here are some tips to help:

◎ **Keep your body warm.** A cold body means cold hands, so layer up and wear a hat.
◎ **Warm your gloves.** Pop them on the radiator before you head out: it's harder to warm hands up once they're cold.
◎ **Experiment with gloves.** Look for gloves which block the wind and try different brands. Mittens rather than gloves can help. Some gloves have battery-powered warmers, and don't forget re-useable hand warmers that can be heated in the microwave.

My hands get so cold and numb with Raynaud's that I can't get my door key in the lock when I get home and I've been near to tears asking a passer-by to open my energy bar mid-run. I'm on tablets now and I use a base liner and Little Hotties hand warmers inside my over-mitts, which even kept my fingers warm during the Genghis Khan ice marathon.   Lucja Leonard, ultra-runner, traveller and adventurer www.runningdutchie.org

◎   **Use liners.** Thermal, silk, cotton or even silver are fabrics used for gloves and liners. Adding that extra layer will trap air and improve insulation.

See your GP if: you have Raynaud's but are struggling with its frequency and severity; medications are available for severe symptoms ▪ you have Raynaud's and other symptoms alongside it such as joint pain and swelling or fatigue.

Varicose veins

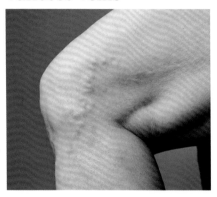

Enlarged, lumpy and often unsightly veins on the legs are called varicose veins. They can be inherited from your parents (thanks mum) but they can also appear in pregnancy, if you're overweight and if you sit or stand for hours on end. The blood travelling in the arteries reaches the feet without any difficulty, but its journey back up to the heart, in the veins is a slow one. Like traffic, the blood flow slows up when it meets an obstruction – for example, a pregnant belly can squash the veins as they enter the pelvis. You know you're in for a traffic jam when three lanes reduce to one on a busy motorway! Similarly, if cars start turning round and trying to go the wrong way down a one-way street, traffic chaos ensues and no one goes anywhere. This is the same picture that develops inside your veins when the valves fail; they usually ensure blood travels in one direction only. You get a 'backing up' of blood, resulting in swollen veins. They're a bluish colour because the blood inside was on its way back to the heart to get more oxygen. Once blood is enriched with oxygen in the lungs it turns back to that familiar 'blood red'.

Exercise helps prevent varicose veins by boosting circulation. When you're active your calf muscles contract and this acts as a pump, helping the flow of blood on its journey through your lower legs. If you have to stand still for a long time, simply rising up and down on your toes frequently will help, as will flexing your feet backwards and forwards when sitting at your desk. Using exercise to help keep your weight in the normal range will lower your risk of varicose veins. Once varicose veins are there exercise unfortunately won't help them to go away. Most people won't need any treatment though; support tights or compression stockings can help prevent throbbing, and elevating your legs after a long day on your feet helps too. If your veins are particularly painful or you have associated skin problems such as itching or ulcers, then there are a variety of procedures you can have to clear them. Very unsightly veins can affect your confidence, but treatment for cosmetic reasons is not available on the NHS and you might choose to have a procedure done

privately. Unfortunately, there's always a risk they'll come back. Varicose veins can bleed heavily when they're knocked so if you're doing contact sports and this happens press firmly on the vein (preferably with a clean cloth or dressing) and lie down on the ground with your leg in the air. If the bleeding isn't stopping, get medical assistance.

See your GP if: your veins are causing you a lot of pain or bleed frequently
▪ you have skin changes such as itching or a rash with your varicose veins.

Headaches

Headaches are common and can certainly stop us exercising. Exercise can both help and trigger headaches so it's worth taking the time to look at them in a bit more detail.

TENSION HEADACHES

Tension headaches are the most common type of headache. We've all felt that pressure and tightness around the sides and front of our head. They're caused by a huge number of things including tiredness, stress and bright lights. They usually only last a few hours and if you know what's causing yours, you can take steps to ease it or take a painkiller if your usual tricks don't work.

MIGRAINE

Migraine is often thought of as a type of headache but in reality it's much more than that and frequent, severe migraines can have a huge impact on all areas of your life. The headache during a migraine can be intense, and it's often accompanied by other symptoms such as nausea, vomiting and visual changes. Alterations in the way you perceive sounds and smells and a strong sensitivity to light are also features of migraine. Attacks can last from several hours to three days and can be severe enough to mean that all you can do is lie still in bed.

Up to a third of people who suffer with migraines experience an 'aura' before the pain of the headache starts. This might be a change in their vision, such as zig-zag lines appearing, an odd smell or a tingling sensation in their face or body. Auras usually last less than an hour and aren't always followed by a headache.

Migraines make my training quite inconsistent. Some days my head hurts too much to even want to move and other days I feel sick and dizzy; obviously I can't exercise when I'm feeling like that. I was taking daily medicine to prevent attacks, but they gave me side effects, so now I'm trying to reduce attacks by cutting out certain foods.   Christina Laidlaw, runner, swimmer, cyclist, climber and knitter

Establishing triggers for your migraines is key to minimising the frequency and severity of attacks. It helps to keep a diary if the causes are not obvious. They can vary from hormonal fluctuations to certain food types, and computer screens to too much caffeine. Like tension headaches, exercise can help or trigger migraines.

Exercise can help: Regular exercise can help you cope with the stresses of everyday life. A chance to quite literally 'clear your head' can mean you're more relaxed, less tense and have fewer migraines and tension headaches. Exercise can also help you to get a good night's sleep and reduce headaches caused by tiredness.

Exercise can trigger: Being dehydrated or hungry can set off a headache, so can exercising in very cold or hot weather. Depending on what activity you do you may find that your posture when you exercise creates tension across your neck and shoulders; cycling or running long distances are prime examples. Sudden strenuous exercise, especially if you don't exercise regularly can be a trigger for headaches.

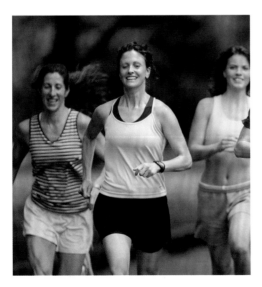

PREVENTING HEADACHES FROM EXERCISE

Prevention is always better than cure, so trying to spot and prevent your headache triggers is important. Dehydration and low blood sugar levels can be avoided by making sure you drink plenty of fluids and consume enough fuel for your activity. If you've been exercising for over an hour, make sure you eat something within 30 minutes of stopping. Relaxing your neck and shoulders, intermittently stretching and altering your posture will prevent tension building up. Bright sunlight can be avoided with sun hats and glasses and wear clothes made from technical fabrics to make sure you don't overheat. Gradually building up the intensity of your exercise and warming up well can help too.

TREATING HEADACHES

Common sense will tell you that if you know what's triggered your headache the first thing to do is to correct it, whether that be rehydrating or getting out of bright light. Heat applied across the back of your neck or on your forehead can ease discomfort, and a neck and shoulder massage relaxes tense muscles. Sometimes going out for some gentle exercise in the fresh air will help. For a tension headache, if you need to take painkillers then paracetamol or anti-inflammatories like ibuprofen are the best option. Migraine treatment is slightly different. It's best to take painkillers as soon as you feel a migrainous headache starting, rather than let it build up. You can use paracetamol and ibuprofen or aspirin, but if these aren't effective then see your GP to discuss the use of a medication called triptans, which work well in combination with paracetamol or anti-inflammatories. You might also need to ask about anti-sickness medications if nausea or vomiting are a feature of your migraine. Medications that are soluble or in liquid form will work more quickly, which is often key in preventing the progression of a migraine. If you're having two or more migraines a month and they're interfering with your daily life for three days or more, speak to your GP about preventative treatments which are taken daily to keep migraines away.

EXERCISE-INDUCED HEADACHES

Any sudden, severe headaches that come on when you're exercising at high intensity need to be checked urgently by a doctor. The fear is that a blood vessel in the brain may have burst, leading to conditions like a sub-arachnoid haemorrhage where blood leaks onto the surface of the brain. These are rare types of stroke and they can kill you. They tend to happen to people in their 50s and 60s, and most are caused by swellings called aneurysms on the blood vessels in your brain. High blood pressure, excessive alcohol and smoking are risk factors for subarachnoid haemorrhages. Aneurysms can burst and leak if you strain hard, so holding your breath whilst lifting a very heavy weight could be a trigger. Call 999 if this happens to you. Exercise-induced headaches are not always due to such a serious cause, but this needs to be excluded.

See your GP if: you're struggling to manage the frequency of your headaches
- you're a migraine sufferer and your normal medications are not working or

> IF YOU HAVE CHEST PAIN AT THE SAME TIME AS PROLONGED PALPITATIONS, YOU SHOULD CALL 999 FOR AN AMBULANCE.

you're needing them frequently ▪ you have a very sudden, very severe headache which makes you feel faint, dizzy or unsteady or makes you vomit. You should call 999 if this is the case.

Palpitations

When you exercise, your heart rate increases because it has to pump blood around your body faster as your muscles call out for oxygen. You can often feel the thump of your heart in your chest but if the beat is particularly fast, strong or irregular then it's called a palpitation. It's normal to get palpitations if you're anxious or scared; they're common around the menopause too.

Every now and then your heart can feel as if it's 'missing a beat'. What's actually happening is that the beat is a little early and there's then a pause waiting for the next one. These are known as ectopic beats and the heart soon catches up with itself. Stress, caffeine and alcohol can cause ectopics and a racing heart (tachycardia), so it's sensible to reduce these if you're experiencing palpitations.

If palpitations only happen occasionally, settle within a few seconds and you don't experience any other symptoms with them, they're most likely harmless. Sometimes, however, palpitations are a sign that all's not well. Heart muscle contracts (squeezes) in response to electrical impulses that pass through its muscle cells. If the pattern of the impulses becomes uncoordinated the heart might beat in an irregular fashion, too quickly or too slowly. Atrial fibrillation (AF) is the most common cause of a persistent irregular pulse. AF needs monitoring and medical treatment due to the increased risk of stroke associated with it.

Dehydration, thyroid problems and anaemia are other common conditions that might cause palpitations.

See your GP if: you're getting palpitations most days ▪ you feel sick, dizzy or short of breath with your palpitations ▪ your palpitations are happening frequently and taking more than a few minutes to resolve ▪ you experience chest pain or tightness with your palpitations ▪ you have a pulse that's irregular or seems to jump around ▪ you have other symptoms such as weight loss or a tremor of your hands.

Chapter 16

LONG-TERM MEDICAL CONDITIONS

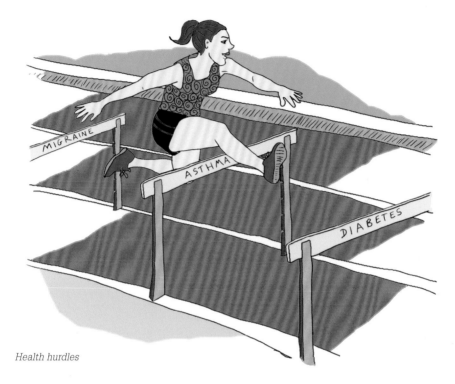

Health hurdles

Sometimes ongoing medical conditions are a minor inconvenience, but at other times they rule and restrict your life. Your confidence to exercise can be severely knocked and you can feel uncertain or afraid as to how much you should be pushing yourself. Everyone with a long-term medical condition will benefit from exercise, and with the right advice and support you should be able to take part and enjoy being active whenever you want.

Cardiovascular disease

Everyone knows that exercise improves your cardiovascular fitness – the health of your heart and blood vessels. What you might not know is that cardiovascular disease is responsible for 10 per cent of female deaths every year in the UK, and that by exercising regularly you can reduce the risk of dying from a cardiovascular event (this includes heart attacks and strokes) by up to a third. If you already have cardiovascular problems, exercise forms an important part of your treatment. It's never too late to start; exercise

A ONE-OFF BP READING IS NOT ALWAYS A TRUE REFLECTION OF YOUR BP, ESPECIALLY IF IT'S TAKEN IN A GP CLINIC. BP READINGS CAN BE FALSELY HIGH IN A CLINIC SETTING; WE CALL THIS 'WHITE COAT SYNDROME'.

will improve the health of your heart and blood vessels whatever your age.

BLOOD PRESSURE

Blood pressure (bp) is quite simply the measure of the pressure in your blood vessels. A bp reading consists of two numbers. The first is called the systolic value and this is the maximum pressure in your blood vessels, when your heart is contracting and pumping. The second number is the diastolic value, which is the minimum pressure in your system, when your heart is resting between beats. Bp is measured in millimetres of mercury (mmHg) and is presented as systolic/diastolic. For example, if your bp is 120/60 the maximum pressure in your blood vessels is 120mmHg and the minimum is 60mmHg.

What's normal?   A bp of 140/90 or below is normal, but the optimum bp sits around 120/80 or lower. If you have other medical problems such as heart disease, diabetes or kidney damage, your ideal bp may be lower and your GP or nurse can advise you. If your bp is higher than 140/90 (either or both numbers) you might have high blood pressure and you'll need some further tests to confirm it. This involves taking home bp measurements or wearing a bp monitor that will take recordings throughout the day and night so your doctor can see what the values are during your day-to-day life. The higher your bp is, the more damage it will do.

Hypertension   High bp is called hypertension and it leads to heart disease, strokes, kidney damage and early death, so it's important to spot and treat. You're more at risk of

Bp machines

Have your blood pressure checked at least every five years. You don't need to see your GP to do this. Lots of pharmacies offer this service and screening services pop up in shopping centres and supermarkets. You can buy your own monitor too; the British Hypertension Society have a list of machines that have been validated for use at home.

hypertension as you get older; it's estimated that half of people over 60 have high bp. Other risk factors include being overweight, being inactive, smoking, a family history of hypertension, excess salt or alcohol in your diet and being of African-Caribbean origin.

EXERCISING REGULARLY IS A GREAT WAY TO REDUCE YOUR RISKS OF HYPERTENSION, BUT YOU NEED TO KEEP IT UP TO CONTINUE TO BENEFIT FROM IT.

Exercise and blood pressure When you exercise, your bp goes up. Your muscles crave oxygen and there are more waste products to dispose of. In response, your heart pumps more forcefully and frequently, causing a rise in the systolic pressure. Interestingly, your diastolic pressure doesn't change much. If you continue to exercise at a comfortable intensity, then the systolic pressure might reduce a little from those higher levels at the start. When you stop, your systolic bp falls to 10-20mmHg below its normal value and may stay there for several hours, even as long as 24 hours in some people.

Exercising regularly will help to prevent and treat hypertension. It's one of the first steps to take if you're diagnosed with mild or moderate hypertension. The heart is a muscle, and with regular training it becomes stronger and more efficient. Larger volumes of blood will be pumped with less effort, reducing the pressure in the system. As your fitness improves, your resting pulse rate (the speed of your pulse when you wake in the morning and before you get out of bed) will reduce and your bp will lower. As muscles grow they require a larger blood supply and new small blood vessels called capillaries grow in the muscle to supply this. Other blood vessels enlarge too, due to

Safety notes

Whilst exercise is an important first step in treating high blood pressure there are a few things to bear in mind. The American College of Sports Medicine (ACSM) advises that if your bp is 180/105 or higher then you shouldn't exercise until it's been stabilised with medication. If you've been diagnosed with hypertension check with your GP whether there are any restrictions for you. It's obviously sensible to start exercise gently and build up. Vigorous activity should be avoided until your blood pressure is under control. See the 'Safety Checklist' at the end of the chapter for more advice on how to exercise safely with a medical condition.

Weight lifting and high blood pressure

A mixture of aerobic exercise and strength training is ideal for maintaining and achieving a healthy bp. While strength training with heavy weights, your bp increases more than it does with other types of exercise, so you shouldn't lift heavy weights if you have uncontrolled bp. It's important to learn how to breathe properly so you can lift without holding your breath, and you should also avoid doing lots of exercise with your arms above your head, as both of these things increase bp.

hormonal triggers and nerve pathways. More and larger blood vessels effectively means that your blood volume is more 'spread out' and the pressure is reduced. With regular exercise you can expect to reduce your bp by approximately 5mmHg, which may be enough to stop you needing medication. Exercise also helps to lose excess weight; being overweight contributes to high bp.

Hypotension Let's consider what happens at the other end of the spectrum too. If your bp is less than 90/60 it's classed as low. It's called hypotension, and it's more common in women than men. It's usually harmless but it can make you feel dizzy or faint, particularly if you stand up too quickly after stooping, sitting or lying. Watch out if you bend over mid-exercise to tie up a shoelace or jump up after floor-based exercises. You also need to take care when you stop exercising. If you stop suddenly, the increased blood flow that your muscles have demanded during vigorous exercise pools in your legs rather than reaching your brain. This can make you feel very unsteady or even pass out. Warming down slowly will reduce the likelihood of this happening. If you have hypotension, try adding a little extra salt to your diet and make sure you're always well hydrated. If you feel faint, lie on the floor, preferably with your legs elevated (it doesn't matter how silly you look), or sit on the ground with your head between your knees.

EXERCISE TO REDUCE CARDIOVASCULAR RISK

As well as high blood pressure, smoking, high levels of bad cholesterol, obesity and diabetes can also put you at risk of cardiovascular disease (CVD). All of these factors make the build-up of fatty deposits in the lining of arteries called atheroma more likely. Like scale inside pipes, atheroma narrows and hardens arteries (atherosclerosis) and impairs blood flow. If blood clots form on these deposits the artery can become completely blocked, which leads to a heart attack or a stroke. Exercise can help improve

When I was 60, I had two heart attacks within two weeks out of the blue. I knew that I was overweight and avoiding exercise after a not-very-successful hip replacement, but coronary heart disease? It was the shock I needed to kickstart a serious diet and exercise regime. Neither would have worked without the other, and both required a lot of discipline, but I was doing it to stay alive and regain some quality of life. As I began to lose weight it was easier to increase my walking distance; I just went a little further each time. I had more puff, even on the hills surrounding our village. I was given a pedometer and tracking my distance has been really motivating. When I go to our local town I'll park the car in the furthest car park from the market and carry my groceries in a backpack. I jump at the chance to run upstairs and fetch something. It all adds up! Two years on I've lost over 50 lbs and I'm maintaining the loss. I no longer have to take all the cardiac drugs as my cholesterol and blood pressure have improved so much. My general mobility is so much better and I'm even told I look 10 years younger. It's been worth the effort; I've got my life back! Sarah-Ann C, 62, retired chiropodist

all of these risk factors – yes, even smoking; if you're physically active you're more likely to give up smoking. Having a family history of CVD also increases your risk. You're classed as having a strong family history if your father or brother was diagnosed with CVD under the age of 55 or your mother or sister was diagnosed under 65. If this is your story, see your GP for a cardiovascular risk assessment before starting vigorous exercise. You can't alter your genetics, so it's important to focus on the things you can change. If you've been diagnosed with cardiovascular disease already, it's still just as important to exercise regularly to reduce your risks of further problems.

SUDDEN CARDIAC DEATH

We've all seen the tragic headlines when someone dies whilst competing in sport. Whether it's during a football match or near the finish line of a marathon, it makes you wonder what your own risks are and it can send out the message that exercise is bad for you. Take running a marathon as an example. If we look at research published in 2012 it might offer some reassurance. Eleven million runners were studied over 10 years and only 42 died from a cardiac arrest during their race; that's approximately one person in 259,000. Most of the deaths were in male runners and were due to hypertrophic cardiomyopathy (HOCM) and coronary heart disease.

> EXERCISE HELPS TO INCREASE THE LEVELS OF GOOD CHOLESTEROL IN YOUR BLOOD WHICH PREVENTS ATHEROMA DEVELOPING IN YOUR ARTERIES.

Sudden cardiac death (SCD) in young people (under 35 years of age) is most likely to be caused by inherited conditions called cardiomyopathies. HOCM is the most common of these, affecting one in 500 people. In this condition the heart wall is thickened. Sometimes symptoms of breathlessness, chest pain and palpitations, occur but it can also cause sudden death with no warning. Many sporting organisations routinely screen their young athletes for HOCM. The organisation Cardiac Risk in the Young (CRY) works hard to offer support to people affected by SCD and promotes and develops screening programmes and medical research. The website (listed at the back of this book) is a great source of information if you have any concerns about this topic. It highlights, however, that screening will not prevent all deaths, as there are certain cardiac conditions that are undetectable on testing.

Deaths during sport due to coronary heart disease are often in those who were unaware they had the condition. It's rare under the age of 30 and more likely if you have other risk factors such as a strong family history. See the section on exercise to reduce cardiovascular risk earlier in this chapter.

Ultimately, exercise is good for your heart health and helps you to live longer, but if you have an underlying heart condition then exercise can make death from this more likely. If you have a family member who had a sudden, unexplained death, there may be screening options available to you and you should discuss this with your GP. Whatever event you're participating in you should train properly by gradually increasing the frequency, intensity and length of your sessions.

Cardiac rehabilitation

Cardiac rehabilitation classes are the ideal way to get the support and expertise you need to return to exercise safely and confidently after heart problems. Heart attacks, heart surgery or insertion of pacemakers are all reasons you might need to consider rehabilitation. You can be referred to classes directly from the hospital or via your GP. You can find out more information through the British Heart Foundation and locate your nearest class via maps.cardiac-rehabilitation.net

HOW MUCH IS TOO MUCH?

The honest answer is we really don't know. There may come a point at which exercise starts to do more harm than good, but what that level is remains unclear and it'll be different for each individual. We know that long-term endurance athletes have a higher risk of atrial fibrillation (AF) where the heart beats in an irregular pattern, leading to an increased risk of stroke. We also know from studies that there are some changes to the right side of the heart and the presence of chemicals, which may represent heart muscle damage, in the blood of endurance runners after a race. Within a week most of these changes fully reverse but in some of the most highly-trained athletes they're longer term. It's possible that if you repeatedly, excessively stress the heart you might develop some scarring of the heart muscle (myocardial fibrosis) which affects its function and causes irregular heart rhythms. To keep things in perspective, consider a study published in the British Journal of Sports Medicine in 2014 which followed elite (male) athletes, including those competing in endurance sports, over 50 years and found they lived five to six years longer than the other healthy men they were compared to. More research needs to be done, but heart damage certainly isn't something that should concern those of us enjoying recreational activity with sensible training plans and adequate rest. Not doing enough exercise is a bigger risk to our health.

Respiratory conditions

ASTHMA

Leading charity Asthma UK report that 4.3 million adults in the UK are currently receiving treatment for asthma; that's one in 12 adults, and it's more common in women than men. Asthma is a long-term condition where the small airways tighten and become swollen and clogged with mucous in response to anything that irritates them. This blocks the movement of air and causes shortness of breath, coughing and wheezing. It's understandable that doing exercise and asking your lungs to work harder might make anyone affected by asthma feel nervous. Being active, however, is essential for good health and there's no reason why well-controlled asthma should stop you exercising. The perfect example of this is Paula Radcliffe, an athlete with asthma, who needs no introduction and proves that performance at the highest level is possible.

Tips for exercising with asthma

Avoid triggers – Viruses, pollen, pollution, cold air and chlorine can all trigger a flare-up of asthma symptoms. To minimise pollen exposure, follow the tips in the section on exercising with hay fever. Urban routes will be better than rural ones when pollen counts are high and keeping the windows closed in the gym will help too.

Pollution levels are higher near busy roads and queuing traffic, so head to green spaces. If cold air is a trigger, avoid outdoor exercise on really chilly days or cover your nose and mouth with a scarf to warm the air you inhale. Try an air-conditioned gym on very hot days if the heat affects you. Chlorine levels in swimming pools vary and pools which use other techniques such as ozone to sanitise the water often have lower chlorine levels.

Anticipate – If asthma is interfering with your exercise and you need to stop and use your 'reliever' inhaler, try having a couple of puffs of it 15–20 minutes before you begin. You can also try this trick on a chilly day if cold air is your trigger. Always carry your 'reliever' inhaler with you when you exercise, even if you don't think you'll need it. Don't forget that if you struggle with asthma during hay fever season then taking a daily antihistamine might help to keep your symptoms under control.

Adapt – Above all, you need to be flexible. You might have to adjust your activity plans according to your environment and asthma control, sometimes swapping to a lower-intensity activity or resting completely. It's important to listen to your body and stop if you're wheezing, coughing, have a tight chest or can't talk. If you've had an asthma flare-up and been unable to exercise, it's best to restart gradually to gauge how you feel.

Breathing exercises

Learning to breathe in a way that's efficient and maximises your lung volume seems an obvious thing to do. There are many breathing techniques such as the Buteyko Breathing Technique and the Papworth method, which are designed to help with asthma and other breathing disorders. Individual trials have shown they reduce asthma symptoms and improve quality of life but a Cochrane review, which assesses all the available evidence on a topic, was carried out in October 2013 and it couldn't come to any reliable conclusions. This is clearly an area needing larger and better quality trials. Remember, breathing techniques should be used alongside and not as a replacement for any prescribed medication.

Ask – Ideally your asthma control should be so good that you rarely need to use your 'reliever' inhaler. If this isn't the case, or if asthma is interfering with your ability to exercise, you need to ask for help from your asthma nurse or GP. You may need to move up a rung on the asthma treatment ladder and increase your daily 'preventer' treatment. You can also ask for an action plan so you know what steps you should take if you feel your asthma is deteriorating.

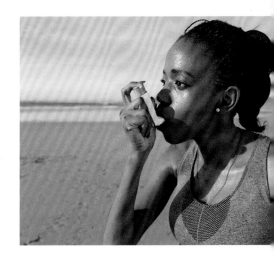

EXERCISE-INDUCED ASTHMA

Many people with asthma, particularly if it's longstanding or poorly controlled, find exercising a struggle and shortness of breath, coughing and wheezing can force them to stop and use their inhaler. There are some people, however, who don't have any day-to-day problems with asthma and the only time they're ever affected is when they exercise. This is sometimes called exercise-induced asthma but it's also known as exercise-induced bronchospasm (EIB). EIB better reflects the fact that there aren't asthma symptoms at any other time but when exercising the airways (bronchi) spasm and narrow, restricting air movement. EIB is particularly common in winter sports, due to the cold, dry air, and in vigorous endurance sports like cross-country running. The symptoms can start during exercise or up to 10 minutes after stopping. They tend to stop after about half an hour but can linger for up to 24 hours. EIB is treated like asthma, with 'reliever' medication taken prior to exercise. If this doesn't work, your doctor may consider using regular 'preventer' medications. What's most important is that you seek help and don't let this stop you exercising.

Asthma and hormones

Asthma can vary with your hormones. Symptoms can flare up just before or during your period, when you're pregnant and around the menopause too. Adapt your exercise plans and talk to your nurse or GP about a change to your treatment if this is happening to you.

See your GP if: you have an unexplained cough ▪ you frequently cough, wheeze or get a tight chest when you exercise ▪ you use your 'reliever' inhaler more than twice a week ▪ your asthma symptoms are interfering with exercise.

COPD

Another common breathing disorder is chronic obstructive pulmonary disease (COPD), which affects around three million people in the UK. COPD includes the conditions emphysema and chronic bronchitis, and it tends to affect people over 40 years of age. The biggest cause of COPD is smoking, and stopping is the single most important thing you can do for your health if you have COPD. It's a progressive disease which means it gets worse, and the airways are permanently damaged and narrowed. The symptoms can be similar to those of asthma and include shortness of breath, wheezing, coughing and too much mucous. Your GP will make the diagnosis of COPD based on your description of how you feel, examining you and a lung function test called spirometry. Treatment for COPD aims to relieve symptoms and prevent chest infections which are common. The airway narrowing is fixed and cannot be opened up as effectively as the reversible narrowing in asthma.

Exercise and COPD If you have COPD you might feel nervous about exercising and making yourself feel more breathless. Because of this, many people with COPD do very little exercise and this is a tragedy because there are many proven, major benefits. Classes called pulmonary rehabilitation are available all over the country and provide structured exercise programmes and education for those affected by breathing disorders. They're an ideal way to gain confidence and improve your fitness in a safe environment. You can ask your nurse, GP or chest specialist to refer you to your local class.

Lung disease and osteoporosis

Medications for lung diseases like asthma and COPD often include treatment with steroids. Regular use of large doses of steroids can increase your risk of osteoporosis. Couple this with the fact that many people with breathing difficulties are less active than they need to be for good bone health, and you can see why there's a potential for weak bones and fractures. It's extra important to exercise regularly to offset these issues. Turn to Chapter 7 to read more about osteoporosis and exercise.

Specialist opinion

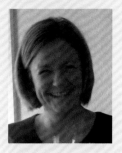

DR JENNIFER HELM, CONSULTANT IN RESPIRATORY MEDICINE AT
BLACKPOOL FYLDE AND WYRE NHS FOUNDATION TRUST, LOVES
TRAVEL, GREAT FOOD, RUNNING AND LONG WALKS

I encourage all my patients with respiratory conditions to
exercise; the physical benefits include stronger breathing muscles,
better lung capacity and weight loss, as well as positive effects on
mental wellbeing. This means people with asthma or COPD have more 'reserve' to fight off
and recover from infections, and feel generally better and more positive day to day. I
reassure them that feeling a little out of breath when exercising is normal, and won't cause
harm. It's important that the type of activity is something they enjoy and that amount of
exercise is built up very gradually over weeks and months. No-one should miss out on the
positive effects of exercise just because they have a chronic chest condition.

If you have COPD and exercise regularly you will:

- slow the progression of your disease;
- be less likely to be admitted to hospital because of your COPD;
- improve your feelings of breathlessness;
- improve your quality of life;
- live longer.

Diabetes

You're probably familiar with the term diabetes and know that it means high blood
sugar, but when we start talking about different types of diabetes, many people feel less
knowledgeable. Over 3.5 million people in the UK have diabetes and seven million more
are at high risk of developing it. The World Health Organisation estimate diabetes
affects over 382 million people worldwide. Diabetes can be a major barrier to exercise,
but exercise is vitally important in treating and preventing it. Let's have a look at the
different types of diabetes and see where exercise fits in.

WHAT IS DIABETES?

The body's main source of energy is glucose, which you get from the food you eat. Your
body likes to keep your blood sugar levels as even and steady as possible. When you

eat, your blood sugar levels rise, causing insulin to be released from a gland called the pancreas (close to your stomach). Insulin causes glucose to move from the blood into your cells and this lowers your blood glucose. When the cells have sufficient glucose the rest is stored as glycogen in your muscles and liver or as fat. It can then be released from these stores when your blood sugar levels dip between meals.

If you have diabetes, you have less insulin and your blood glucose levels are high because the glucose doesn't move into your cells. There are two types of diabetes:

Type 1 diabetes   This most commonly starts in childhood or adolescence. It's one of those autoimmune conditions that keep popping up throughout this book, where the body starts attacking itself. The target here is the cells in the pancreas that make insulin. If you have type 1 diabetes you aren't making insulin and you have to monitor your blood glucose levels and replace the insulin by injecting it into yourself.

Type 2 diabetes   This type of diabetes usually develops later in life and is more common if you're overweight. It affects about one in 17 people in the UK but that's the tip of the iceberg, as many people are undiagnosed. The pancreas does make insulin in type 2 diabetes but it either doesn't make enough or the body is 'insulin-resistant' and doesn't respond properly to the insulin that's present. Initially, type 2 diabetes is treated with lifestyle changes such as an improved diet and regular exercise. For many this will be sufficient to return glucose levels to normal. The next step is the use of medication to lower glucose levels; there are many different types and the commonest one is metformin, a tablet which is taken daily. You might need to move onto other tablets or medications given by injection, including insulin.

WHAT'S A NORMAL GLUCOSE LEVEL?

◎   Blood glucose is measured in millimoles per litre (mmol/L).

◎   A glucose reading less than 4 mmol/L is low.

◎   A normal glucose reading before you eat is 4–7 mmol/L.

◎   A glucose reading above 7 mmol/L when you've fasted or a random blood glucose above 11 mmol/L suggests diabetes.

◎   If your doctor arranges a glucose tolerance test for you, you'll be given a big sugary drink to consume and your blood will be checked two hours later. A level above 11 mmol/L confirms diabetes.

◎   A test called HbA1c is also used to detect and monitor diabetes. It gives an idea of what your blood sugar levels have been over the previous eight to 12 weeks, rather than just giving a snap shot at one point in time. An HbA1c of over 48 mmol/L (also known as 6.5%) is classed as diabetic. An HbA1c of 42–37 mmol (6.0 to 6.4%) indicates you're at high risk of developing diabetes and need to take urgent action to improve your lifestyle and stop the onset of diabetes.

HYPERGLYCAEMIA AND HYPOGLYCAEMIA

These terms are often misunderstood. Hyperglycaemia means that the level of glucose in the blood is generally too high. This gives the symptoms of diabetes, which include feeling tired, thirsty, losing weight and needing to pass lots of urine. Hypoglycaemia means glucose levels are too low. This is not a symptom of diabetes, it's a result of the treatment. If you have type 1 diabetes and the insulin you've taken is too much for the amount you've eaten or the activity you're doing, then your blood glucose can fall below normal levels. How this affects people varies, but it might make you feel lightheaded, sweaty or shaky. You might feel really hungry, moody or confused. Hypoglycaemia (a 'hypo') needs to be treated as soon as possible by eating glucose tablets or drinking a sugary drink to get your sugar levels up quickly.

COMPLICATIONS OF DIABETES

In the short term, very high levels of glucose can make you unwell and can even be life-threatening. Over the long term, diabetes makes you five times more likely to have a heart attack or stroke. It damages blood vessels, leading to blindness, kidney damage and poor circulation in your feet. It also damages the nerves in skin, which causes numbness in hands and feet and a risk of skin ulcers. There are risks for you and your baby if you get pregnant too. It's crucial to have proper monitoring and treatment if you have diabetes of any type.

Feet, exercise and diabetes

If you have diabetes you need to be obsessive about looking after your feet. Diabetes affects both the blood and nerve supply, making the skin on your feet very vulnerable. Infections are more likely and harder to treat. Loss of sensation in the feet is common, so you might not even know you have an area that's rubbing, or that a piece of grit has got inside your shoe. When you've finished exercising take off your shoes and socks, wash and dry your feet and check them over thoroughly. Look for areas of pressure and breaks in the skin, and get advice from a chiropodist if you're concerned. Well-fitting shoes and socks are vital.

DIABETES AND EXERCISE

It's really important to exercise regularly if you have diabetes. Here's why:

◎ Exercise can help you get better control of your blood sugar; being active regularly increases your sensitivity to insulin.

◎ Exercise helps you to normalise your weight. It might reduce or stop the need for medication if you have type 2 diabetes and are overweight and manage to lose some.

◎ Diabetes puts you at higher risk of heart disease and stroke, and we know that exercise helps to reduce this risk by reducing blood pressure and cholesterol levels.

◎ Exercise can help you cope with the stress of having a long-term health problem.

WHAT TYPE OF EXERCISE SHOULD YOU DO?

There's no reason for you to limit your choice of activity if you have diabetes. It's important to take part in a range of different types of exercise. Being sedentary puts you at an increased risk of type 2 diabetes. Getting up every 20 to 30 minutes and having a walk around for a couple of minutes can help to reduce this risk. Moderate or vigorous intensity exercise (aerobic exercise), where you're working your heart and lungs, will help prevent against the cardiovascular complications of diabetes like heart attacks and stroke, but strength training to build muscle is important too. A study in 2007 looked at 251 adults with type 2 diabetes and found that improvements in blood sugar levels were greatest when general fitness training and strength training were combined. This is backed up by a huge study which followed 32,000 men in the USA over 18 years. It concluded that at least two and a half hours of weight training a week can reduce the risk of developing type 2 diabetes by 34%. Doing aerobic training for the same length of

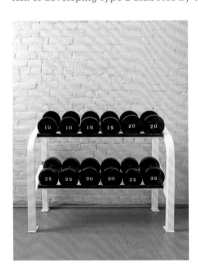

time reduced the risk by 54% but the greatest reduction in risk was by 59% in the men that were doing a combination of the two, compared to those that were doing nothing. Obviously, this study was in men, and it's not clear what type or intensity of weight training was being done, but it's likely that the benefits would be similar in women. Following the recommended guidelines for exercise that include aerobic and strength exercises is a sensible way to get the health benefits of exercise. Check back to Chapter 1 for a reminder of these guidelines.

Specialist opinion

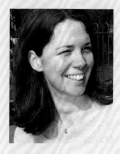

DR JENNIFER BEYNON, CONSULTANT DIABETOLOGIST AT UNIVERSITY HOSPITAL OF SOUTH MANCHESTER, MUM OF THREE, LOVES TO SKI AND KAYAK

I'm strongly in favour of exercise for my patients. I've only ever seen positive effects from it, including weight loss, medication and blood pressure reduction and improved mood and energy levels. However, it does require planning and extra monitoring. Always start exercise gently and monitor your sugars frequently during and after exercise until you're confident of the effect it has. Speak to your diabetes team for encouragement and support.

TYPE 1 DIABETES

Check your blood sugar and test your urine before exercise. If your blood sugar is over 14mmol/L or there are ketones in your urine, don't exercise. Instead take a correction dose of insulin and consider exercising later. Always carry some form of hypo treatment with you.

Your risk of hypoglycaemia increases during and immediately after exercise and up to 24 hours afterwards. You can either eat more carbohydrate (roughly 10–20g for every hour of exercise) or reduce your insulin before and after exercise to balance this. It's essential to monitor your blood sugars frequently. If you're starting something new or increasing your intensity, monitor them every 30-60 minutes, from an hour before the exercise to three to four hours afterwards. How you balance the extra carbohydrate and reduction in insulin will depend on the time of the day, intensity and duration of the exercise and the timing of your next meal. See page 243 and ask your local diabetes team.

TYPE 2 DIABETES

It's generally safe to exercise with type 2 diabetes. If you're taking insulin or sulphonylureas such as gliclazide discuss your exercise plans with your diabetes team. Whatever your medication is, it's still important to check your blood sugar before exercise; it may be safe to exercise at a starting level above 14mmol/L if you have type 2 diabetes, but discuss this with your team. Remember exercise may help you lose weight and make you more sensitive to insulin. Both of these may lead to more hypoglycaemic episodes, possibly unrelated to exercise; if you notice this you'll probably need a reduction in your medication.

Don't exercise within 24 hours of a hypoglycaemic episode and remember that alcohol increases hypoglycaemia risk so exercising after a night out requires extra vigilance.

I was diagnosed with type 1 diabetes aged eight. I was reluctant to accept it at first, but within a few weeks I was testing and injecting myself. I've always been active. As a child I did every sport I could fit into my week, from horse riding to swimming, netball to trampolining and football to cross-country. My diabetes consultant was fantastic in supporting me to continue with my exercise. I now go to the gym frequently and I've played netball for my college, county and university, as well as a number of clubs at a competitive level. The balance between my sport and diabetes has been tricky over the years, particularly trying to combat hormones! Diabetes UK care events have been especially helpful and each time I've learnt new ways to manage my diabetes in order to do what I wanted. Moving to an insulin pump has given me tighter control around food and exercise and my bloods have improved.

I've always ensured someone from my team is aware of my diabetes and certainly don't hide it, yet people do seem to forget I'm diabetic as I simply get on with it and do the same as everyone else. It's never been an issue with any of my teammates; their response is positive as they admire my approach to not letting my diabetes determine what I do and don't do.   Jennifer Bartley, 26, primary school teacher

I was diagnosed with type 2 diabetes about five years ago. I was devastated. It felt like everything was going wrong with my health. I was angry, depressed, scared and obstinate. I cried when I heard what changes I had to make to my diet, but I did it. I cut down on carbs and ate more fruit and veg, and I lost over two and a half stone. I also stopped smoking; I'd smoked 25–30 cigarettes a day for 40 years. I knew I had to increase my activity so I bought a bike and started cycling with the dog. This progressed to cycling to work, which was a 14-mile round trip. I walked more too and started swimming three times a week. I started to enjoy exercise and felt happier and less stressed. I also wasn't as tired or lethargic as I had been. The exercise definitely helped to bring my blood sugar levels down. I'm really fed up at the moment as I'm waiting for a knee operation. My weight has gone up a bit and I've had to start a new diabetes tablet. I'm desperate to get back to the swimming and cycling as soon as I can.   Wiggy, 57, lives in Hedon, mother of one child and two dogs

Epilepsy

In epilepsy, sudden and abnormal electrical activity fires off in the brain. The result is a seizure, also known as a fit. How it affects you is dependent on which areas of your brain are involved. It can range from brief moments of inattention caused by a small focus of electrical activity to total body seizures, where the impulses spread more generally through the brain tissue. Over half a million people in the UK have epilepsy, which means they've had repeated seizures. There can be an underlying cause, such as a brain injury, but for the majority there's no reason for it. It can start at any age, but most commonly begins in childhood or after 60. Anti-epileptic medications are used to calm brain activity and control seizures. Over time some seizures stop and don't return, but for many, epilepsy is a long-term condition affecting daily life.

Everyone should be able to enjoy exercise, and in the past people with epilepsy have often been discouraged from being active for fear of triggering seizures or putting themselves at risk. Now, however, the trend is thankfully towards encouraging exercise because of the major health benefits it brings.

TRIGGERS FOR SEIZURES

Everyone's experience of epilepsy is very different; you need to become an expert in your own condition. There's always a risk of sudden unexpected seizures, but this is rare if you have controlled epilepsy. Learning to avoid or minimise your triggers will help you exercise safely. Missing your medications will obviously reduce your control and if you're unwell with an illness it can make seizures more likely too. Seizures can be more frequent at certain times of the month or even the time of day, so it makes sense to avoid these times when you're planning your exercise. Other common triggers relevant to exercise include dehydration, low blood sugar and extreme heat. These can become very important if you're taking part in endurance events. Keeping hydrated by drinking frequently and learning how to manage your fuelling is crucial. Going to high altitude rapidly should be avoided, as that can trigger a seizure in some people with epilepsy. Tiredness and stress can be a trigger too. You sometimes need to look at the bigger picture to get the best control. There are a small minority of people who find that intense strenuous exercise will trigger a seizure and they have to keep to low-intensity activities. Many people with epilepsy, however, find that exercise actually helps to control seizures which are triggered by stress, tension and lack of sleep.

POTENTIAL RISKS WITH SEIZURES

You can exercise freely with well-controlled epilepsy, but if your epilepsy isn't fully controlled and you have occasional seizures, you need to take some extra precautions to keep yourself and those around you safe when you exercise. This is especially important when you know one of your trigger factors might be relevant, such as your stress levels or missed medication. If you're cycling, walking or running then it's sensible to avoid busy roads or routes like canal paths where you're exercising right next to water. Never swim alone, regardless of how well controlled your epilepsy is, and if you think a seizure is a possibility in a public pool, it's a good idea to tell the lifeguard so they can take prompt action if you get into difficulty. If your epilepsy is poorly controlled, it's not advisable to climb or be in charge of belaying someone else. Horse riding, sailing and skiing are other sports that might pose a risk to you if you have a seizure. It's wise to wear a helmet for any activity where head injury is possible. It's all a balance of risks, and once you know your own epilepsy well you can decide whether a sport is safe for you. If you're in doubt, discuss it with your specialist nurse or doctor. Have a look at the 'Safety tips' that follow for more advice.

I began exercising because I felt sluggish and unfit and wanted to get into shape; I chose running. My epilepsy wasn't the worst it's been when I started, but it wasn't fully controlled. I signed up to the Great South Run and then got a place in the marathon. Since I started exercising I've found a marked improvement in my epilepsy. Running allows me to clear my head, so the mental stresses slip away. Sleep deprivation has always been a big trigger for me, so although exercising makes me physically tired, my sleep quality is better and I've found this has really helped. Running long distances has encouraged me to eat really well and view food as fuel, which has made a difference too. I honestly believe exercising regularly has helped control my epilepsy. It's also amazing to know my body can do this despite having this condition. Faye Waddams, 30, London

Safety checklist

If you have a medical condition, make sure you follow these steps when you exercise.

◎ Always tell someone where you're going and when you plan to be back.

◎ It's ideal to exercise with a friend who understands your health problem and knows how to help you.

◎ Always carry a mobile phone and don't forget to add a number to your contacts under ICE (In Case of Emergency). Some phones have an emergency feature accessible without a password from the front screen so that important health information is available.

◎ Consider wearing medical jewellery or carrying medical ID to let others know about your health in an emergency.

◎ Let instructors or coaches know about your condition and explain what they need to do if you become unwell.

◎ Fill in the details on the back of your competitor bib when you're entering events. Marshall and medics who help you will look there for vital information.

◎ Always start any new exercise plans slowly and build up gradually. Warm up and cool down properly too.

◎ Stop and rest if you feel unwell in any way, for example if you feel dizzy, have chest pain or difficulty breathing.

◎ Take your medications regularly and always carry any 'just in case' medications such as inhalers or dextrose tablets with you when you exercise.

◎ Always be a little cautious about exercise if you've had a change in your usual medication, as it might upset your normal control or give you unexpected side effects.

◎ Be flexible with your exercise plans and adapt them if you don't feel 100 per cent or if your medical condition has been unstable.

◎ Speak to your GP or nurse if you are at all unsure about any symptoms, treatment or suitability of an activity.

Anti-epileptics and exercise

In order to control your seizures you may need to take daily medication. All medications can have side effects, and common ones with anti-epileptic drugs are weight gain and tiredness. Exercise can help you to control your weight and also improve feelings of fatigue. Long-term, high doses of some anti-epileptic medications can also cause an increased risk of osteoporosis (thinning of the bones). This is largely a concern if you also have very reduced mobility, little exposure to sunlight or inadequate calcium in your diet. Keeping active will help to minimise your risk of osteoporosis; read more about this in Chapter 7. It's also wise to bear in mind that the blood levels of some anti-epileptic medications can be affected by exercise so if you're about to embark on a new intense training plan, have a chat with your doctor first.

Chapter 17

FINDING THE TIME AND THE MOTIVATION

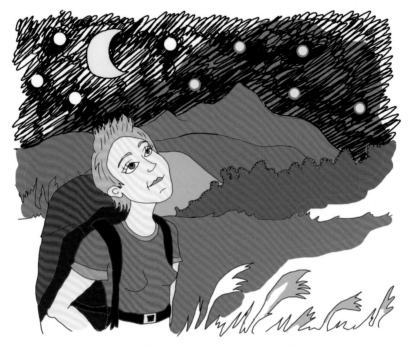

The only person you're competing against is yourself

Two of the biggest barriers to exercise are time and motivation. Squeezing exercise into your already jam-packed day is a major challenge and it's easy to ruin all your good intentions. Life has a habit of throwing other things at you to knock you off course too. Many women with busy jobs and family lives, however, are keeping active, regularly, and loving it. Finding that exercising gives you energy, health and an inner strength and confidence is a wonderful discovery. Here are some tips and tricks of mine along with some from wonderful women who are out there doing it.

Creating time

We all have 24 hours in each day, but some of us are better at time management than others. You need to get clever and grab small windows of opportunity; remember that just a 10-minute block of exercise is beneficial. Imagination and delegation are key: seven-year-olds can load and unload dishwashers if you teach them how, older kids can

Strange though it sounds, I find I manage to fit more into my life when I'm training for a marathon. You just have to be so organised. I follow a training plan and run at least four times a week. I rarely miss a session. If I do, I feel really guilty. I tend to do my long runs at the weekend when my husband's around with the kids. In the week when I'm working, I'll plan when I'm running in advance. If I can't find enough time, I run to or from work to make sure I fit it in. I've even been known to use a day's leave to make sure I get an important long run done. People often ask me how I manage to juggle a full-time job, three kids and running. But once you get into the rhythm of marathon training, it's very doable. In fact, I miss it when it's over. The training gives me so much more energy. I love the space and thinking time. Plus, it gives me a goal, something to aim for, not to mention all those endorphins...   Sophie Raworth, BBC newsreader, presenter, mum of three and long-distance runner

hang out washing, and delegating your supermarket shop to a delivery service will gain you hours, not minutes. Watch out for time-wasters like social media, where hours literally vanish! Time spent looking for things or making last-minute dashes to the shops can be recovered by generally being more organised. The book *Time Management for Manic Mums* by Allison Mitchell is full of tips and techniques to help make every day run more smoothly but also to free up time for you to follow your dreams. I don't know how I would've found the hours required to train for my first marathon without Allison's book.

Making exercise part of your normal daily activities is easier than setting aside specific time to do it. Choose to walk whenever possible, for example; brisk walking will boost your heart rate and actually save you time. Cycling to work, taking the stairs instead of the lift and getting off the bus early are all suggestions you've heard before, but they do work. Look for every opportunity to make the day harder: squats while the kettle boils, sit-ups on the floor whilst watching TV with the kids; it's amazing how active you can be within your normal day if you try.

It's not selfish to claim this time for yourself. Being fit and healthy will help you be more effective in all areas of your life. Prioritise that time, make sure it happens regularly and guard it ferociously. Enlisting the help of others who understand can give you more options, so devise plans with friends and family to make it happen. Alternatively, get them joining in too and find activities to enjoy together.

I was intimidated by the guidelines of doing 150 minutes' exercise a week and was moaning to my husband about it when he quietly asked me, 'Why don't you just walk from your office to the station instead of getting the bus?' I decided to try it out and realised that it took just five minutes longer to walk as the bus was always stuck in traffic. I did it for a week and realised I was now just 25 minutes short of the 150-minute target. Then I began walking to the office in the mornings too and bingo – I'd actually exceeded the target by 100 minutes! And the extra time cost was only 10 minutes a day – plus I discovered a lot of interesting shops along the way. Lisa Williams, 48, copywriter

All I wanted to do was to go for a quick run, but with three small children at home I couldn't see a way to manage it. A friend who also runs suggested we did a relay and she brought her three children round to my house. We put them all in the garden to play and I looked after all six for half an hour while she ran and then we swapped over. The kids had a great time, we both got our run and a coffee and catch-up afterwards; it set me up for the day. Kris Parkinson, mum of three, cycles, runs and kayaks

Goal setting

It's wonderful to have dreams and easy to set targets, but it's very difficult to realise and reach them. One of the main problems is that a goal is often overwhelming and it can feel unachievable, especially as you're trying to reach it alongside your normal life. This is particularly true if you're feeling stressed, anxious or low in mood, when even the act of putting on your trainers and heading out of the door can be too much to contemplate. It's important to set goals though, because working towards them motivates you and reaching them makes you feel good.

The secret of reaching a goal is to break it down into small steps. The steps can be tiny, as miniscule as they need to be to be achievable. Just keep asking yourself what you need to do to make the next step happen. Let's take an example:

'I'm feeling really down, unfit and stodgy. I want to do some exercise so I feel fitter and better about myself. I used to like going out on my bike but it's been in the garage for ages with a broken chain that I don't know how to fix and I really haven't got time to sort it out. Even if it was working I don't think I'd get far as I'm so unfit and I'm worried about going on my own in case I get lost or have a mechanical problem.'

Clearly this woman needs to get her bike fixed, get riding again and it looks like doing that within a group would help allay her concerns.

Let's break it down into steps:

1 Search online for a bike repair shop.

2 Phone the repair shop and book a slot.

3 Drop bike off.

4 Pick bike up.

5 Go out on bike for five minutes to see how it feels.

6 Go out on bike for 15 minutes.

7 Go out on bike for 30 minutes.

8 Search online for local Breeze network (women-only bike rides) or similar.

9 Send an enquiry to local team leader to find out when the next beginners ride is.

10 Get kit and bike ready for ride.

11 Go on ride for one hour with the group.

Each of these steps is manageable and won't take very long. Each one is moving her closer to her target. Writing them all on the calendar, not more than one a day and ticking them off as she does them, will make her feel she's achieved something that day. Within three weeks she'll have reached a target that seemed impossible. If she'd gone straight for the 'I'm going on a long bike ride' option, she'd have fallen at the first hurdle because it wasn't achievable. She'd have felt like a failure and it would've put her off trying again.

This 'small steps' principle can be applied to any task or target, however small or large. Just keep asking what you need to do next and before you know it you'll be at the end. Running marathons, decorating a bedroom, completing a work project; just keep breaking it down until there's a step small enough for you to do. If you don't manage a step, maybe it's because it was too big or perhaps you need to ask someone for help to achieve it. Just keep moving forwards. As your confidence grows you can be more daring with your targets and start to realise some of your dreams.

Finding motivation

Once you've found windows of time and got started, the next problem is maintaining your enthusiasm and motivation. How many times have you started a new 'fitness regime', only to find it's all fizzled out after a month? There are lots of ways to keep that fire burning. Here's my advice followed by tips from world champion Chrissie Wellington and top motivational expert Kim Ingleby.

FINDING SOMETHING YOU LOVE

You're not going to keep something up long term if you don't enjoy it. Exercise isn't just about running, cycling and swimming. Think fencing, golf, canoeing and squash; the possibilities are endless. Sport England's hugely successful This Girl Can campaign has been a wonderful reminder that all women can be active and you need to be brave and step out of that comfort zone sometimes. Stop caring what you look like and just go out and have fun. Persuading a friend to go with you can boost your confidence. You can get so much support and motivation from others. It might just be one person to drag you out of the front door, a team sport or a whole community, like parkrun. You might, however, prefer individual sports where you purely rely on yourself. Experimenting and finding what works for you takes time and often a bit of courage.

MIXING IT UP

Even when you've found something you enjoy, you can get stale after a while. If your motivation is waning and you find you've been skipping sessions, just mix it up a bit. Try something different, perhaps just for one day, perhaps for a few months. It's great for your body to be doing a range of activities to work all your different muscle groups, so you'll find you get stronger too.

USING TECHNOLOGY

Although technology is one of the things that's made us more inactive as a society, it's also one of the solutions to help us become more active. Pedometers and health apps offer motivation by tracking your steps and activity. Uploading your activity means you can share your efforts and injects a bit of competition. Writing blogs or sharing your goals and progress on social media not only helps to keep you focused but provides a support network of others in the same situation. You can get endless advice and

My advice to other women would be to find an activity you enjoy; you might need to try a few things before you hit your favourite. It'll be worth it and you'll be amazed at how much confidence it gives you, how many friends you'll make and how welcoming the sporting world is! I was so nervous going back to the gym after decades away and yet everyone was so kind and supportive. Do it for yourself, don't compare and don't be intimidated by people who have more skill or experience than you. Jo Moseley, rower and founder of healthyhappy50.com

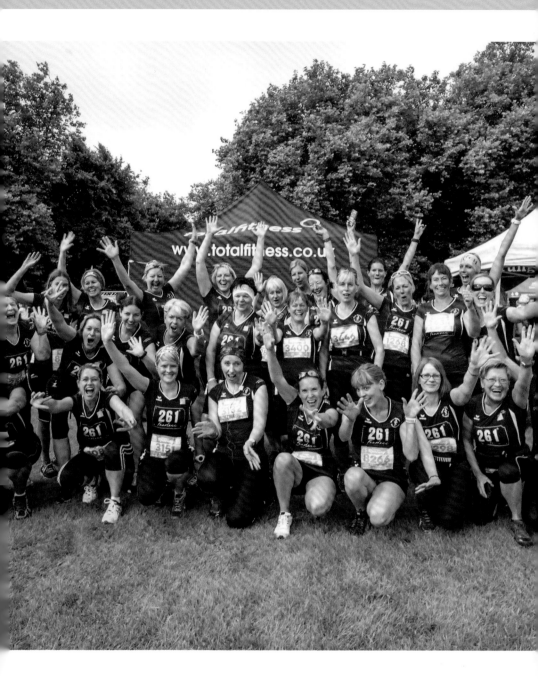

encouragement at any hour of the day or in any moment of weakness on Twitter forums such as UKSportsChat or Facebook communities like Run Mummy Run and 261 Fearless. Social media links you to others with common goals and interests, which stops you boring ambivalent friends and relatives! Use it to your advantage, keep an open mind and give it a go, ask a tech savvy friend to help you get started.

I went to a boxing class for the first time last night, it was ace! I didn't feel judged, I just did what I could and gave everything a go. I'm sure I'll feel it in my muscles tomorrow. It was fabulous to just do something totally different! Angie Miller, mum of two in Derby, hates rude people

After my second baby I was struggling to keep to fixed commitments and could never get to my evening running club, as my husband was rarely home from work by then. I missed chatting to like-minded people, especially of the running variety, so I started a small Facebook group of women to connect with. Run Mummy Run now has over 20,000 women members. We provide motivation, support and a sense of belonging to our ladies. Ability is irrelevant, we just salute every runner who's making the effort to lace up their trainers. Creating this secure, non-judgmental environment allows our members to use their running to grow in confidence and feel happy in many other aspects of their lives. Leanne Davies, founder of Run Mummy Run (www.runmummyrun.co.uk). A mother of two with a passion for running and all the good it brings

I took up golf when I retired as a way to keep active and help my high cholesterol levels. I never imagined that I would go on to play for my county and win individual and team trophies! Going out on a golf course for the first time can make you feel exposed and vulnerable, and many women don't have the confidence to do it. I helped with some taster lessons and a 10-week academy for women to try golf. Watching ladies find their feet and develop a love for the game has been such an amazing experience. It's opened up opportunities for them all as they now feel able to play on courses all over the country. It's really made me want to get better too! Lyn Bond, 64, golfer, grandmother to four

HELPING OTHERS

Helping others to exercise might not be an obvious way to motivate yourself, but it's a really powerful one. My personal experience starting a running group in my village has been one of my major motivators over the past two years. Supporting other women and watching them flourish has given me as much pleasure as my own running.

Specialist opinion

Who better to advise us on staying motivated than Chrissie Wellington, winner of the Ironman Triathlon World Champion title an incredible four times. An ironman involves a 2.4-mile swim, a 112-mile bike ride followed by a marathon, in that order, without stopping. That takes some motivation to train for and complete, let alone be the best in the world at!

Of all the questions I'm asked, the most common has to be, 'How do you stay motivated?' People tend to assume that pros are blessed with unwavering and limitless drive, determination and vitality; that we never feel lethargic or lazy, and that the thought of donning a 'onesie' and performing a sofa-slump never crosses our minds. This couldn't be further from the truth. I, like the rest of the human race, suffer from motivational ebbs and flows. The key is that we learn to recognise, prevent, manage and mitigate mojo-malaise and stop it from totally derailing us from the pursuit of our goals. Make your goal clear, realistic yet slightly ambitious too. Close your eyes and picture yourself as being strong, confident, and successful – standing at the finish line with your loved one in one hand and a post-race doughnut in the other. Do it – close your eyes – visualise! You're only as powerful as your mind! Starting is often the hardest part. So, do just that. Start. Be adaptable; focus on what you can do. Perfection is doing the best you can in the context of your life. Be inspired by music. Be inspired by words. Be inspired by others. If they can, you can. We all suffer from motivational ebbs and flows. It's normal, it's natural, but it's also under our control. We can crack the case. Make today something really special. Be the very best that you can be!

CELEBRATE SUCCESS

It helps to celebrate your successes at each stage along your journey. Every step counts, and working towards a treat or simple pleasure really does make a difference. It might be a trip to the hairdresser, a soak in the bath or a large piece of chocolate cake, it doesn't matter. When you smash that final target and conquer your goal then get out the flags, crank up the music and bask in the glory! Celebrate with friends and family: you deserve it and you'll inspire them to set challenges for themselves too. Don't underestimate the power that your own actions have to motivate others. You can then move on to planning your next goal.

Specialist opinion

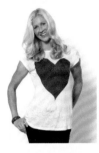

TIPS FROM A PROFESSIONAL MOTIVATOR

If you're very serious about reaching a goal you might turn to a professional for guidance. I asked award-winning and leading UK mind and body expert Kim Ingleby from www. energisedperformance.com and www.kimingleby.co.uk to share her motivational secrets and strategies. Here are her top ten tips.

1 **Become really clear on your motivation and your intention.** Write down all the reasons why you're going to achieve your goal (get fitter, lighter etc) and next to the reason, why this is important to you and how this makes you feel. Then highlight the top three motivators and pin them somewhere to remind you of your goal daily and to help when motivation is low.

2 **Make a plan that works for you and stick to it.** Write down three mini goals you're going to achieve each week to allow you to reach your big goal, and prioritise them in your diary. This will allow you to feel in control of your goal. Every time you achieve a mini goal, stick a gold star in your diary, or put £1 in a money box. It sounds simple but these reward systems help to boost motivation and keep you on track.

3 **Make yourself accountable with two people.** Once you have a clear goal and time frame and your motivation is clear and positive, choose two people to tell what you're planning to do in detail, how you would like to feel and how they could support you. By sharing things with people you're much more likely to achieve your goal, and enjoy the process. Choose people who will be positive and encouraging in their support to you.

4 **Keep a feel-good diary.** Buy a journal and write down three things you did well each day, and one thing you would do differently. You'll notice if you have a limiting pattern, and can do something to change this to ensure you achieve your goal.

5 **Stop self-sabotaging and comparing.** It's hard to start to think positively about yourself if you've always been negative, but try to be aware of making unhelpful comparisons with others around you. Start with, 'I'm safe and I'm OK'. This will allow you to move away from your limiting thoughts and towards a positive state. The more you think about how you would like to feel and be, the easier it will become. The trick is to start with something easy like, 'I'm OK'.

6 **Be flexible and listen to your body.** Be kind to yourself. You have your plans and goals but it's important to be flexible if there are times of stress or you're unwell. Allow these

days to pass, but put a date in your diary when you'll get back on track. Make sure you eat healthy, nutritious, fresh food, hydrate well and sleep deeply for positive results. If your body is feeling good, it'll be easier to increase your confidence and mental strength in sport.

7 **Model behaviour and results from people who inspire you.** A really important tip is to choose two or three people who inspire you and 'act as if' you had those qualities. For instance, you may admire confidence, self-respect and happiness as qualities in different people. Watch how they behave, listen to what they say, and try to imagine what it would feel like to be in their body – then 'act as if' you did have these qualities. It can be a famous athlete, a celebrity or a friend – just a person who represents a quality you would like more of. Focus on being your best on the day, and let go of comparisons with others.

8 **Have a positive word for the day (or four!)** Decide on the main feelings or a mantra you could benefit from having in your thoughts for the day, for example, 'Today I will become leaner, fitter and stronger', 'I will be my best on the day' or 'Confidence and motivation'. Use these words and mantras every day to reinforce moving towards the person you want to become. Combined with this, remember to stand tall and be proud of the person you are. Breathe in what you want to feel, think and do and breathe out what you don't want to feel, think and do.

9 **Create a vision board.** Take a big sheet of coloured paper or a pin board and write in the middle 'What do I need to do to achieve my goal?' Then write down around it all the things you need to do, all the excuses you might come up with, plus a solution to overcome them (this is key). Cut out photographs, places, people and stick them on the board too. You could do this as a blog, Pinterest board or video blog. Each time you review, write or post, it will enhance your motivation towards achieving what you want.

10 **Be proud of you and have fun.** Remember the power of positive thoughts, consistent little steps and kindness to yourself. One day wrong is fine; just get on track the next day. It takes 21 days to change a habit, and 21 days to set a new habit.

During this time you may feel a bit uncomfortable, but if you've got your support team and your motivation's really clear you'll be able to ride through the uncomfortable place to an even better, happier one, and achieve your goals in sport and life.

So start each day with the intention of being the very best version of yourself, be authentic, be you and have the courage to dare to go for it.

End note

Exercise opens up a whole new world to us. Not only can it make us feel fitter, stronger and empowered but it brings opportunities: the chance to make friends, laugh, share, travel and explore. For some, like me, it may even bring a change of direction in life and work. We need to be brave, make bold choices and embrace these opportunities. I hope this book has helped you to break down your health barriers and get yourself sorted so you can enjoy all that an active life has to offer you. If it has I'd love you to let me know. Tweet me @JulietMcGrattan or visit my blog www.drjulietmcgrattan.com.

Useful websites

Chapter 1: Why bother?

www.nhs.uk

English Federation of Disability Sport

www.efds.co.uk

Chapter 2: Periods

Diary-doll pants www.diarydoll.com

Polycystic ovaries www.verity-pcos.org.uk

Moon Cup menstrual cups

www.mooncup.co.uk

Endometriosis support

www.endometriosis-uk.org

Premenstrual syndrome www.pms.org.uk

Chapter 3: Breasts

Breast biomechanics research

http://www.port.ac.uk/department-of-sport-
and-exercise-science/research/breast-
health/

Breast cancer prevention and research

www.breastcancernow.org

Help and support for breast cancer

www.breastcancercare.org.uk

Chapter 4: Pregnancy

Pregnancy www.emmasdiary.co.uk

SPD and pelvic joint pain in pregnancy

www.pelvicpartnership.org.uk

Chapter 5: New Mums

Breastfeeding

www.breastfeedingnetwork.org.uk

Pre and postnatal depression support and
advice www.pandasfoundation.org.uk

Chapter 6: The Pelvic Floor

Urinary symptoms and incontinence

www.bladdermatters.co.uk

www.pelvictoner.co.uk

www.incostress.com

www.evbsport.com

www.squeezyapp.co.uk

Chapter 7: The Menopause and Beyond

Menopause Matters

www.menopausematters.co.uk

National Osteoporosis Society

www.nos.org.uk

Women's stories of the menopause

http://www.healthtalk.org/peoples-
experiences/later-life/menopause/topics

Chapter 8: Mental Health

Mental health information and support

www.mentalhealth.org.uk

www.mind.org.uk

www.moodcafe.co.uk

www.anxietyuk.org.uk

Online self help and CBT

www.moodgym.anu.edu.au

www.llttf.com

www.beatingtheblues.co.uk

www.moodjuice.scot.nhs.uk

The Samaritans for advice and support
with a free 24-hour telephone helpline

www.samaritans.org

Telephone 116 123 from the UK and
Republic of Ireland

Eating disorders www.b-eat.co.uk

Chapter 9: The Digestive System

The IBS network for information and
advice about IBS and applications for a
toilet card www.theibsnetwork.org

CORE - For information including fact
sheets and leaflets about all types of
digestive disorders

www.corecharity.org.uk

Coeliac disease www.coeliac.org.uk

Bladder and Bowel Foundation for
information, support and applications for
a toilet card

www.bladderandbowelfoundation.org

Macmillan for advice and support for those affected by all types of cancers and for applications for a toilet card
www.macmillan.org.uk
For disability advice and support and applications for a toilet key
www.disabilityrightsuk.org

Chapter 10: Skin
Hyperhidrosis support group
www.hyperhidrosisuk.org
National Eczema Society www.eczema.org
Psoriasis Association
www.psoriasis-association.org.uk

Chapter 11: Tired all the Time
British Thyroid Foundation
www.btf-thyroid.org
ME and Chronic fatigue syndrome
www.meassociation.org.uk

Chapter 12: Muscles and Joints
Restless legs www.rls-uk.org
Fibromyalgia Action UK www.fmauk.org
Arthritis Research UK
www.arthritisresearchuk.org

Chapter 13: Common illnesses
www.nhs.uk
www.patient.info

Chapter 14: Common Injuries
www.running-physio.com
www.kinetic-revolution.com

Chapter 15 Common Medical Problems
Allergy UK www.allergyuk.org
Scleroderma & Raynaud's UK
www.sruk.co.uk
The Migraine Trust
www.migrainetrust.org

Chapter 16 Long-Term Medical Conditions
Asthma UK www.asthma.org.uk
British Lung Foundation www.blf.org.uk
British Heart Foundation www.bhf.org.uk
British Hypertension Society
www.bhsoc.org
Diabetes UK www.diabetes.co.uk
Help with balancing diet, insulin and exercise
www.excarbs.com
www.runsweet.com
Cardiac Risk in the Young (CRY)
www.c-r-y.org.uk
Epilepsy Action www.epilepsy.org.uk
Epilepsy Society
www.epilepsysociety.org.uk

Chapter 17 Finding the Time and the Motivation
Breeze bike rides for women
www.goskyride.com/Breeze/Index
Parkrun www.parkrun.org.uk
UKSportsChat www.uksportschat.co.uk
Run Mummy Run www.runmummyrun.co.uk
This Girl Can www.thisgirlcan.co.uk
261 Fearless www.261fearless.org

Recommended reading

Jackson, Lisa. *Your Pace or Mine?: What Running Taught Me About Life, Laughter and Coming Last.* Summersdale (2016)

Kessel, Anna. *Eat Sweat Play: How Sport Can Change Our Lives*, Macmillan, London (2016)

Macdonald, Christina. *Run Yourself Fit: Simple Steps to a Healthier You.* Vie (2016)

McAndrew, Nell and Waterlow, Lucy. *Nell McAndrew's Guide to Running.* Bloomsbury Sport (2015)

Mitchell, Allison. *Time Management for Manic Mums: Get Control of Your Life in 7 Weeks.* Hay House UK (2012)

Murray, Dr Andrew. *Running Your Best.* lulu.com (2015)

Parker, Dr Claire and Gray, Sir Muir. *Sod Sixty!: The Guide to Living Well.* Bloomsbury Sport (2016)

Percy, Kate. *Go Faster Food: Over 100 energy-boosting recipes for runners, cyclists, swimmers and rowers.* Vermillion (2009)

Switzer, Kathrine. *Marathon Woman: Running the Race to Revolutionize Women's Sports.* Da Capo Press Inc (2009)

Wellington, Chrissie. *A Life Without Limits.* Constable (2013)

Whalley, Susie. Jackson, Lisa. *Running Made Easy.* Collins and Brown (revised edition 2014)

Whyte, Professor Greg. *Bump It Up: The dynamic, flexible exercise and healthy eating plan for before, during and after pregnancy*, Bantam Press, London (2016)

References

I've read hundreds of scientific papers to make sure my advice to you is sound and up to date. I don't want to bore you with all of the references but here are some of the main ones which you can go to for more information.

Chapter 1

Department for Transport. National Travel Survey: England 2013
http://www.gov.uk/government/uploads/system/uploads/attachment_data/file/342160/nts2013-01.pdf [Accessed 2015]

Department of Health. UK physical activity guidelines
http://www.gov.uk/government/publications/uk-physical-activity-guidelines [Accessed 2015]

Public Health England. 'Everybody active every day'
http://www.gov.uk/government/uploads/system/uploads/attachment_data/file/374914/Framework_13.pdf [Accessed 2015]

US Department of Health and Human Services. Physical Activity Guidelines Advisory Committee Report 2008
http://health.gov/paguidelines/report/pdf/committeereport.pdf [Accessed 2015]

Chapter 2

Amercian College of Sports Medicine. 'Information on The Female Athlete Triad'
http://www.acsm.org/docs/brochures/the-female-athlete-triad.pdf [Accessed 2016]

Hewett, T.E. Zazulak, B.T. Myer, G.D. (2007), 'Effects of the menstrual cycle on anterior cruciate ligament injury risk: a systematic review'. *The American Journal of Sports Medicine*, 35(4):659-668

Mountjoy, M. Sundgot-Borgen, J. Burke, L. Carter, S. Constantini, N. Lebrun, C. Meyer, N. Sherman, R. Steffen, K, Budgett, R. Ljungqvist, A. 'The IOC consensus statement: beyond the Female Athlete Triad—Relative Energy Deficiency in Sport (RED-S)'
http://bjsm.bmj.com/content/48/7/491.full.pdf+html [Accessed 2015]

NICE. Clinical Knowledge Summaries 'Dysmenorrhoea'
http://cks.nice.org.uk/dysmenorrhoea [Accessed 2015]

NICE. Clinical Knowledge Summaries 'Menorrhagia'
http://cks.nice.org.uk/menorrhagia [Accessed 2015]

RCOG (2014) Green-top Guideline No. 33. 'Long-term Consequences of Polycystic Ovary Syndrome' *http://www.rcog.org.uk/globalassets/documents/guidelines/gtg-33-pcos-2014.pdf* [Accessed 2015]

Royal College of Obstetricians and Gynaecologists. (2007) Green-top Guideline No. 48. 'Management of Premenstrual Syndrome' www.rcog.org.uk/womens-health/clinical-guidance/management-premenstrual-syndrome-green-top-48

Chapter 3

Amit, G. (2011), 'Breast Pain'. BMJ Clinical Evidence http://www.ncbi.nlm.nih.gov/pmc/articles/PMC3275318/ [Accessed 2015]

Mills, C. Lomax, M. Ayres, B. Scurr, J. (2015), 'The movement of the trunk and breast during front crawl and breaststroke swimming'. *Journal of Sports Sciences*, 33(4): 427–436

Risius, D. Milligan, A. Mills, C. Scurr, J. (2015), 'Multiplanar breast kinematics during different exercise modalities'. *European Journal of Sport Science*, 15(2):111–117

Scurr, J. Hedger, W. Morris, P. Brown, N. (2014), 'The prevalence, severity and impact of breast pain in the general population'. *The Breast Journal*, 20(5):508–513

White, J. Scurr, J. (2012), 'Evaluation of professional bra fitting criteria for bra selection and fitting in the UK'. *Ergonomics*, 55(6):704–711

Chapter 4

Artal, R. O'Toole, M. (2003), 'Guidelines of the American College of Obstetricians and Gynecologists for exercise during pregnancy and the postpartum period'. *British Journal of Sports Medicine*, 37:6–12

Centre for Maternal and Child Enquiries (CMACE). (2010), 'Maternal obesity in the UK: Findings from a national project' http://www.publichealth.hscni.net/sites/default/files/Maternal%20Obesity%20in%20the%20UK%20executive%20summary.pdf [Accessed 2015]

RCOG Statement 4 (2006), 'Recreational exercise and pregnancy' http://www.rcog.org.uk/globalassets/documents/patients/patient-information-leaflets/pregnancy/recreational-exercise-and-pregnancy.pdf [Accessed 2015]

Chapter 5

Boyle, R. Hay-Smith, E.J. Cody, J.D. Mørkved, S. (2012), 'Pelvic floor muscle training for prevention and treatment of urinary and faecal incontinence in antenatal and postnatal women'. *Cochrane Database of Systematic*

Reviews, 17;10: CD007471. doi: 10.1002/14651858.CD007471.pub2

The Breastfeeding Network (2002), 'Assessing the evidence: Cracked nipples and moist wound healing' http://www. breastfeedingnetwork.org.uk/wp-content/ pdfs/Cracked_Nipples_and_Moist_Wound_ Healing_2002.pdf [Accessed 2015]

Chapter 6

Bø, K. Talseth, T. Holme, I. (1999), 'Single blind, randomised controlled trial of pelvic floor exercises, electrical stimulation, vaginal cones, and no treatment in management of genuine stress incontinence in women'. *BMJ*, 318 (7182):487–493

Dumoulin, C. Hay-Smith, J. (2008), 'Pelvic floor muscle training versus no treatment for urinary incontinence in women. A Cochrane systematic review'. *European Journal of Physical and Rehabilitation Medicine*, 44(1):47–63

MHRA Regulating Medicines and Medical Devices. (2014), 'A summary of the evidence on the benefits and risks of vaginal mesh repair implants' http://www.gov.uk/government/uploads/ system/uploads/attachment_data/ file/402162/Summary_of_the_evidence_on_ the_benefits_and_risks_of_vaginal_mesh_ implants.pdf

NICE guidelines [CG171] (2013), 'Urinary incontinence in women: management' http://www.nice.org.uk/guidance/cg171

Chapter 7

Asikainen, T.M. Kukkonen-Harjula, K. Miilunpalo, S. (2004), 'Exercise for health for early postmenopausal women: a systematic review of randomised controlled trials'. *Sports Medicine*, 34(11):753–778

Bailey T.G., Cable N.T., Aziz N., Atkinson G., Cuthbertson D.J., Low D.A., Jones H. (2016), 'Exercise training reduces the acute physiological severity of post-menopausal hot flushes'. *Journal of Physiology - London*, 594:657–667

Lethaby, A. Marjoribanks, J. Kronenberg, F. Roberts, H. Eden, J. Brown, J. (2013), 'Phytoestrogens for vasomotor menopausal symptoms'. *Cochrane Database of Systematic Reviews*, 10;12:CD001395. doi: 10.1002/14651858. CD001395.pub4

Leach, M.J. Moore, V. (2012), 'Black cohosh (Cimicifuga spp.) for menopausal symptoms. *Cochrane Database of Systematic Reviews*, 12;9:CD007244. doi: 10.1002/14651858.CD007244.pub2

National Osteoporosis Guideline Group (2014), 'Guideline for the diagnosis and management of osteoporosis in post-menopausal women and men from the

age of 50 years in the UK'
http://www.shef.ac.uk/NOGG/NOGG_
Pocket_Guide_for_Healthcare_Professionals.
pdf [Accessed 2016]

NICE guidelines [NG23] (2015),
'Menopause: diagnosis and
management'
http://www.nice.org.uk/guidance/ng23
[Accessed 2016]

NICE guidelines [CG146] (2012),
'Osteoporosis: assessing the risk of
fragility fracture'
http://www.nice.org.uk/guidance/cg146
[Accessed 2016]

Chapter 8

Cooney, G.M. Dwan, K. Greig, C.A. Lawlor,
D.A, Rimer, J. Waugh, F.R. McMurdo, M.
Mead, G.E. (2013), 'Exercise for
depression'. *Cochrane Database of
Systematic Reviews*, 12;9: CD004366.
doi:10.1002/14651858.CD004366.pub6

NICE guidelines [CG9] (2004), 'Eating
disorders in over 8s: management' http://
www.nice.org.uk/guidance/cg9 [Accessed
2016]

NICE guidelines [CG90] (2009),
'Depression in adults: recognition and
management'
http://www.nice.org.uk/guidance/cg90
[Accessed 2016]

Chapter 9

NICE guidelines [CG61] (2008), 'Irritable
bowel syndrome in adults: diagnosis and
management' http://www.nice.org.uk/
guidance/cg61 [Accessed 2016]

NICE guidelines [CG184] (2014), 'Gastro-
oesophageal reflux disease and
dyspepsia in adults: investigation and
management'
http://www.nice.org.uk/guidance/cg184
[Accessed 2016]

NICE guidelines [NG20] (2015), 'Coeliac
disease: recognition, assessment and
management' http://www.nice.org.uk/
guidance/ng20 [Accessed 2016]

Peters, H.P.F. De Vries, W.R. (2001)
'Potential benefits and hazards of
physical activity and exercise on the
gastrointestinal tract'. Gut, 48:435–439

Public Health England. (2010) 'SACN Iron
and Health Report'
http://www.gov.uk/government/uploads/
system/uploads/attachment_data/
file/339309/SACN_Iron_and_Health_Report.
pdf [Accessed 2016]

Chapter 10

BASHH (2007), 'UK National Guideline on
the Management of Vulvovaginal
Candidiasis' http://www.bashh.org/
documents/1798.pdf [Accessed 2016]

BASHH (2012), 'UK National Guideline for the management of Bacterial Vaginosis' http://www.bashh.org/documents/4413.pdf [Accessed 2016]

Kwok, C.S. Gibbs, S. Bennett, C. Holland, R. Abbott, R. (2012), 'Topical treatments for cutaneous warts'. *Cochrane Database of Systematic Reviews*, 12;9:CD001781. doi: 10.1002/14651858.CD001781.pub3

NICE. Clinical Knowledge Summaries (2013), 'Hyperhidrosis', http://cks.nice.org.uk/hyperhidrosis [Accessed 2016]

NICE. Clinical Knowledge Summaries (2015), 'Tiredness/fatigue in adults' http://cks.nice.org.uk/tirednessfatigue-in-adults [Accessed 2016]

Verdon, F. Burnand, B. Stubi, C.L. Bonard, C. Graff, M. Michaud, A. Bischoff, T. deVevey, M. Studer, J.P. Herzig, L. Chapuis, C. Tissot, J. Pécoud, A. Favrat, B. (2003), 'Iron supplementation for unexplained fatigue in non-anaemic women: double blind randomised placebo controlled trial'. *BMJ*, 326(7399):1124

Chapter 11

Lippi, G. Schena, F. Salvagno, G.L. Aloe, R. Banfi, G. Guidi, G.C (2012), 'Foot-strike haemolysis after a 60-km ultramarathon'. *Blood Transfusion*, 10(3):377–383

Moncrieff, G. Fletcher, J. (2007), 'Tiredness'. *British Medical Journal*, 334(7065), 1221

NICE guidelines [CG53](2007), 'Chronic fatigue syndrome/myalgic encephalomyelitis (or encephalopathy): diagnosis and management' https://www.nice.org.uk/guidance/cg53 [Accessed 2016]

NICE. Clinical Knowledge Summaries (2011), 'Hypothyroidism' http://cks.nice.org.uk/hypothyroidism [Accessed 2015]

Chapter 12

American College of Sports Medicine. (2011), 'Delayed Onset Muscle Soreness' http://www.acsm.org/docs/brochures/delayed-onset-muscle-soreness-(doms).pdf [Accessed 2016]

Bleakley, C. McDonough, S. Gardner, E. Baxter, G.D. Hopkins, J.T. Davison, G.W. (2012), 'Cold-water immersion (cryotherapy) for preventing and treating muscle soreness after exercise'. *Cochrane Database of Systematic Reviews*, Issue 2. Art. No.: CD008262. DOI: 10.1002/14651858.CD008262.pub2

Busch, A.J. Barber, K.A. Overend, T.J. Peloso, P.M. Schachter, C.L. (2007), 'Exercise for treating fibromyalgia syndrome'. *Cochrane Database of Systematic Reviews*, Oct 17;(4):CD003786

Chakravarty, E.F. Hubert, H.B. Lingala, V.J. Zatarain, E. Fries, J.F.(2008), 'Long Distance running and Knee Osteoarthritis. A Prospective Study'. *American Journal of Preventive Medicine*, 35(2): 133–138

Hill, J. Howatson, G. van Someren, K. Leeder, J. Pedlar, C. (2014), 'Compression garments and recovery from exercise-induced muscle damage: a meta-analysis'. *British Journal of Sports Medicine*, 48(18):1340–1346

NICE guidelines [CG177] (2014), 'Osteoarthritis: care and management' http://www.nice.org.uk/guidance/cg177 [Accessed 2016]

NICE. Clinical Knowledge Summaries (2015), 'Restless legs syndrome' http://cks.nice.org.uk/restless-legs-syndrome [Accessed 2016]

Chapter 13

Kreher, J.B. Schwartz, J.B. (2012), 'Overtraining Syndrome: A Practical Guide'. *Sports Health*, 4(2): 128–138

Pedersen, B.K. Toft, A.D. (2000), 'Effects of exercise on lymphocytes and cytokines'. *British Journal of Sports Medicine*, 34:246–251

Chapter 14

Fredericson, M. Wolf, C. (2005), 'Iliotibial band syndrome in runners: innovations in treatment'. *Sports Medicine*, 35: 451–459

Galbraith, R.M. Lavallee, M.E. (2009), 'Medial tibial stress syndrome: conservative treatment options'. Current Reviews in Musculoskeletal Medicine, 2(3):127–133

Kader, D. Saxena, A. Movin, T. Maffulli, N. (2002), 'Achilles tendinopathy: some aspects of basic science and clinical management'. *British Journal of Sports Medicine*, 36:239–249

Lavine, R. (2010), 'Iliotibial band friction syndrome'. *Current Reviews in Musculoskeletal Medicine*, 3(1-4):18–22

NICE. Clinical Knowledge Summaries (2015), 'Plantar fasciitis'. http://cks.nice.org.uk/plantar-fasciitis [Accessed 2016]

NICE. Clinical Knowledge Summaries (2015), 'Shoulder pain'. http://cks.nice.org.uk/shoulder-pain [Accessed 2016]

NICE. Clinical Knowledge Summaries (2015), 'Sprains and strains'. http://cks.nice.org.uk/sprains-and-strains [Accessed 2016]

NICE guidelines [CG176] (2014), 'Head injury: assessment and early management' https://www.nice.org.uk/guidance/cg176 [Accessed 2016]

Chapter 15

Keles, N. (2002), 'Treating allergic rhinitis in the athlete'. *Rhinology*, 40:211–214

NICE. Clinical Knowledge Summaries (2015), 'Migraine' http://cks.nice.org.uk/migraine [Accessed 2016]

Sorace, P. 'Exercising with Allergies and Asthma'. *American College of Sports Medicine. Current Comment* http://www.acsm.org/docs/current-comments/allergiesandasthmatemp.pdf [Accessed 2016]

Chapter 16

Rundell, K.W. Jenkinson, D.M. (2002), 'Exercise-induced bronchospasm in the elite athlete'. *Sports Medicine*, 32(9):583–600

Freitas, D.A. Holloway, E.A. Bruno, S.S. Chaves, G.S.S. Fregonezi, G.A.F. Mendonça, K.M.P.P. (2013), 'Breathing exercises for adults with asthma'. *Cochrane Database of Systematic Reviews* Issue 10. Art. No.: CD001277. DOI: 10.1002/14651858.CD001277.pub3

SIGN guidelines [SIGN 141] (2014), 'British guideline on the management of asthma' http://www.brit-thoracic.org.uk/document-library/clinical-information/asthma/btssign-asthma-guideline-2014/ [Accessed 2016]

NICE guidelines [CG127] (2011),'Hypertension in adults: diagnosis and management' http://www.nice.org.uk/guidance/cg127 [Accessed 2016]

Swedish National Institute of Public Health. (2010), 'Physical activity in the prevention and treatment of disease' http://www.fyss.se/wp-content/uploads/2011/02/fyss_2010_english.pdf [Accessed 2016]

Cornelissen, V.A. Smart, N.A. (2013), 'Exercise training for blood pressure: a systematic review and meta-analysis'. *Journal of the American Heart Association*, 2(1):e004473. doi: 10.1161/JAHA.112.004473

La Gerche, A. Burns, A.A.T. Mooney, D.J. Inder, W.J. Taylor, A.J. Bogaert, J. MacIsaac, A.I. Heidbüchel, H. Prior, D.L. (2012), 'Exercise-induced right ventricular dysfunction and structural remodelling in endurance athletes'. *European Heart Journal,* 33(8):998–1006

Wilson, M. O'Hanlon, R. Prasad, S. Deighan, A. Macmillan, P. Oxborough, D. Godfrey, R. Smith, G. Maceira, A. Sharma, S. George, K. Whyte, G. (2011), 'Diverse patterns of myocardial fibrosis in lifelong, veteran endurance athletes'. *Journal of Applied Physiololgy* 110:1622–1626

Trivax, JE. Franklin, BA. Goldstein, J.A. Chinnaiyan, K.M. Gallagher, M.J deJong, A.T. Colar, J.M. Haines, D.E. McCullough, P.A. (2010), 'Acute cardiac effects of marathon running'. *Journal of Applied Physiology*, 108:1148–1153

Kettunen, J.A. Kujala, U.M. Kaprio, J. Bäckmand, H. Peltonen, M. Eriksson, J.G. Sarna, S. (2015), 'All-cause and disease-specific mortality among male, former elite athletes: an average 50-year follow-up'. *British Journal of Sports Medicine*, 49:893–897

Kim, J.H. Malhotra, R. Chiampas, G.

d'Hemecourt, P. Troyanos, C. Cianca, J. Smith, R.N. Wang, T.J. Roberts, W.O. Thompson, P.D. Baggish, A.L. Race Associated Cardiac Arrest Event Registry (RACER) Study Group. (2012), 'Cardiac arrest during long-distance running races'. *New England Journal of Medicine*, 366(2):130–40

Arida, R.M. Cavalheiro, E.A. da Silva, A.C. Scorza, F.A. (2008), 'Physical activity and epilepsy: proven and predicted benefits'. *Sports Medicine*, 38(7):607–15

National Osteoporosis Society. (2012), 'Anti-epileptic drugs and osteoporosis' https://nos.org.uk/media/1953/anti-epileptic-drugs-and-osteoporosis-december-2015.pdf

Index